Detection, Assessment, Diagnosis and Monitoring of Caries

Monographs in Oral Science

Vol. 21

Series Editors

A. Lussi Bern
G.M. Whitford Augusta, Ga.

Detection, Assessment, Diagnosis and Monitoring of Caries

Volume Editor

Nigel Pitts Dundee

57 figures, 53 in color, and 25 tables, 2009

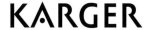

Basel · Freiburg · Paris · London · New York · Bangalore ·
Bangkok · Shanghai · Singapore · Tokyo · Sydney

Nigel Pitts
Dental Health Services and Research Unit
University of Dundee
Mackenzie Building, Kirsty Semple Way
Dundee DD2 4BF (UK)

This volume received generous financial support from Colgate Palmolive Europe.

Library of Congress Cataloging-in-Publication Data

Detection, assessment, diagnosis, and monitoring of caries / volume editor,
Nigel Pitts.
 p.; cm. -- (Monographs in oral science, ISSN 0077-0892 ; v. 21)
 Includes bibliographical references and indexes.
 ISBN 978-3-8055-9184-3 (hard cover : alk. paper)
 1. Dental Caries. I. Pitts, Nigel.
 [DNLM: 1. Dental Caries--diagnosis. 2. Dental Caries--prevention &
control. 3. Health Promotion. 4. Patient Compliance.   W1 MO568E v.21 2009
/ WU 270 D479 2009]
 RK331.D48 2009
 617.6'7--dc22
                                                                 2009016412

Bibliographic Indices. This publication is listed in bibliographic services, including Current Contents®

Disclaimer. The statements, opinions and data contained in this publication are solely those of the individual authors and contributors and not of the publisher and the editor(s). The appearance of advertisements in the book is not a warranty, endorsement, or approval of the products or services advertised or of their effectiveness, quality or safety. The publisher and the editor(s) disclaim responsibility for any injury to persons or property resulting from any ideas, methods, instructions or products referred to in the content or advertisements.

Drug Dosage. The authors and the publisher have exerted every effort to ensure that drug selection and dosage set forth in this text are in accord with current recommendations and practice at the time of publication. However, in view of ongoing research, changes in government regulations, and the constant flow of information relating to drug therapy and drug reactions, the reader is urged to check the package insert for each drug for any change in indications and dosage and for added warnings and precautions. This is particularly important when the recommended agent is a new and/or infrequently employed drug.

All rights reserved. No part of this publication may be translated into other languages, reproduced or utilized in any form or by any means electronic or mechanical, including photocopying, recording, microcopying, or by any information storage and retrieval system, without permission in writing from the publisher.

© Copyright 2009 by S. Karger AG, P.O. Box, CH–4009 Basel (Switzerland)
www.karger.com
Printed in Switzerland on acid-free and non-aging paper (ISO 9706) by Reinhardt Druck, Basel
ISSN 0077–0892
ISBN 978–3–8055–9184–3
e-ISBN 978–3–8055–9185–0

Contents

VII   **List of Contributors**

1   **Introduction.** How the Detection, Assessment, Diagnosis and Monitoring of Caries Integrate with Personalized Caries Management
Pitts, N.B. (Dundee)

15   **Clinical Visual Caries Detection**
Topping, G.V.A.; Pitts, N.B. (Dundee)

42   **Traditional Lesion Detection Aids**
Neuhaus, K.W. (Bern); Ellwood, R. (Manchester); Lussi, A. (Bern); Pitts, N.B. (Dundee)

52   **Novel Lesion Detection Aids**
Neuhaus, K.W. (Bern); Longbottom, C. (Dundee); Ellwood, R. (Manchester); Lussi, A. (Bern)

63   **Lesion Activity Assessment**
Ekstrand, K.R. (Copenhagen); Zero, D.T. (Indianapolis, Ind.); Martignon, S. (Bogotá); Pitts, N.B. (Dundee)

91   **Patient Caries Risk Assessment**
Twetman, S. (Copenhagen); Fontana, M. (Indianapolis, Ind.)

102   **Dentition and Lesion History**
Eggertsson, H.; Ferreira-Zandona, A. (Indianapolis, Ind.)

113   **Assessing Patients' Health Behaviours.** Essential Steps for Motivating Patients to Adopt and Maintain Behaviours Conducive to Oral Health
Freeman, R. (Dundee); Ismail, A. (Philadelphia, Pa.)

128   **Personalized Treatment Planning**
Pitts, N.B. (Dundee); Richards, D. (Stirling)

144   **Background Level Care**
Pitts, N.B. (Dundee)

149   **Traditional Preventive Treatment Options**
Longbottom, C. (Dundee); Ekstrand, K.R. (Copenhagen); Zero, D.T. (Indianapolis, Ind.)

156 Novel Preventive Treatment Options
Longbottom, C. (Dundee); Ekstrand, K.R. (Copenhagen); Zero, D.T. (Indianapolis, Ind.); Kambara, M. (Osaka)

164 Traditional Operative Treatment Options
Ricketts, D.N.J.; Pitts, N.B. (Dundee)

174 Novel Operative Treatment Options
Ricketts, D.N.J.; Pitts, N.B. (Dundee)

188 Recall, Reassessment and Monitoring
Clarkson, J.E. (Dundee); Amaechi, B.T. (San Antonio); Ngo, H. (Singapore); Bonetti, D. (Dundee)

199 Implementation. Improving Caries Detection, Assessment, Diagnosis and Monitoring
Pitts, N.B. (Dundee)

209 Glossary of Key Terms
Longbottom, C. (Dundee); Huysmans, M.-C. (Nijmegen); Pitts, N.B. (Dundee); Fontana, M. (Indianapolis, Ind.)

217 Author Index
218 Subject Index

List of Contributors

B.T. Amaechi
UTHSCSA Department of Community Dentistry
7703 Floyd Curl Drive MC 7917
San Antonio, Texas 78229–3900 (USA)

D. Bonetti
Dental Health Services and Research Unit
University of Dundee
Mackenzie Building, Kirsty Semple Way
Dundee DD2 4BF (UK)

J.E. Clarkson
Dental Health Services and Research Unit
University of Dundee
Mackenzie Building, Kirsty Semple Way
Dundee DD2 4BF (UK)

K.R. Ekstrand
University of Copenhagen
20 Nørre Allé
DK–2200 Copenhagen (Denmark)

H. Eggertsson
Department of Preventive and Community
Dentistry Oral Health Research Center,
Indiana University School of Dentistry
415 Lansing Street
Indianapolis, IN 46202 (USA)

R. Ellwood
Skelton House
Manchester Science Park
Manchester M15 6SH (UK)

A. Ferreira-Zandona
Department of Preventive and Community
Dentistry Oral Health Research Center,
Indiana University School of Dentistry
415 Lansing Street
Indianapolis, IN 46202 (USA)

M. Fontana
Department of Preventive and Community
Dentistry
Indiana University School of Dentistry
Indianapolis, Ind. (USA)

R. Freeman
Dental Health Services and Research Unit
University of Dundee
Mackenzie Building, Kirsty Semple Way
Dundee DD2 4BF (UK)

M.- C. Huysmans
Department of Cardiology & Endodontology
TRIKON: Institute for Dental Clinical Research
University of Nijmegen, PO Box 9101
6500 HB Nijmegen (The Netherlands)

A. Ismail
Maurice H. Kornberg School of Dentistry
Temple University
Philadelphia, Pa. (USA)

M. Kambara
Department of Preventive and Community
Dentistry
Osaka Dental University
Osaka (Japan)

C. Longbottom
Dental Health Services and Research Unit
University of Dundee
Mackenzie Building, Kirsty Semple Way
Dundee DD2 4BF (UK)

A. Lussi
Department of Preventive, Restorative and
Pediatric Dentistry
School of Dental Medicine
University of Bern
Freiburgstrasse 7
CH–3010 Bern (Switzerland)

S. Martignon
Research Centre
Dental Faculty
Universidad El Bosque
Bogotá (Colombia)

K.W. Neuhaus
Department of Preventive, Restorative and
Pediatric Dentistry
School of Dental Medicine
University of Bern
Freiburgstrasse 7
CH–3010 Bern (Switzerland)

H. Ngo
5 Lower Kent Ridge Road
Singapore 119074 (Singapore)

N.B. Pitts
Dental Health Services and Research Unit
University of Dundee
Mackenzie Building, Kirsty Semple Way
Dundee DD2 4BF (UK)

D. Richards
Department of Public Health
NHS Forth Valley
Carseview House
Castle Business Park
Stirling (UK)

D. Ricketts
Dundee Dental Hospital and School
Park Place
Dundee DD1 4HR (UK)

G.V.A. Topping
Dental Health Services and Research Unit
University of Dundee
Mackenzie Building, Kirsty Semple Way
Dundee DD2 4BF (UK)

S. Twetman
Department of Cariology and Endodontics
Faculty of Health Sciences
University of Copenhagen
Nørre Allé 20
DK–2200 Copenhagen N (Denmark)

D.T. Zero
Indiana University School of Dentistry
Indianapolis, Ind. (USA)

Introduction

How the Detection, Assessment, Diagnosis and Monitoring of Caries Integrate with Personalized Caries Management

N.B. Pitts

Dental Health Services and Research Unit, University of Dundee, Dundee, UK

Abstract

This chapter provides an overview of how the detection, assessment, diagnosis and monitoring of caries integrate with personalized caries management. The background includes the continuing burden of preventable disease that dental caries represents on a global scale. Despite this, and evidence that a purely restorative approach will not 'cure' the disease, preventive caries control has been slow to be adopted in many countries. Following a series of initiatives in the last decade, there is now a range of clinical criteria and tools that can be employed to help clinicians plan patient-centred comprehensive and preventively biased care for their patients. At the core is a sound foundation of lesion detection, assessment and diagnosis which, when combined with appropriate patient level risk information and monitoring, enables effective treatment planning. The International Caries Detection and Assessment System (ICDAS) can enable this process. The ICDAS provides clinical criteria and codes, together with a framework to support and enable personalized comprehensive caries management for improved long-term health outcomes. The target audience for this book comprises those with an interest in dental caries and its clinical management; this should in no way detract from the parallel missions in the domains of dental public health, research or education. If progress is to be made in this field, it is important that a compatible series of terms can be shared across the dental domains and across countries. This will ensure better clinical and patient understanding and help facilitate getting research findings into clinical practice in a more efficient way.

Copyright © 2009 S. Karger AG, Basel

Dental caries continues to provide a very sizeable burden of preventable disease on a global scale [1, 2]. A 2009 editorial in *The Lancet* points out that 'oral health is a neglected area of global health and has traditionally registered low on the radar of national policy makers', that dentists prefer 'to treat rather than prevent oral diseases' and 'yet, globally, the burden of major oral diseases and conditions is high. Dental caries is one of the most common chronic diseases worldwide. 90%

of people have had dental problems or toothache caused by caries' [1]. Although the editorial properly focusses on ensuring that other professions also engage in caries prevention as 'good oral health should be everybody's business' [1], there is also much that can be achieved in parallel by the dental profession embracing a more preventive approach to caries management. An earlier *Lancet* review concluded that 'the approach to primary prevention should be based on common risk factors; secondary prevention and treatment should focus on management of the caries process over time for individual patients, with a minimally invasive, tissue-preserving approach' [2].

Despite these clear views, built on evidence and international consensus, and the knowledge that a purely restorative/surgical approach will not 'cure' the disease [3], preventive caries control has been slow to be adopted in many countries. This preventable disease still accounts for many general anaesthetics for children in hospital settings, and decades of restorative work have led many adults to accumulate restorations, more caries and serially repeated restorations. This produces, in many 'developed' countries, cohorts of seniors and older adults with many more retained teeth than their predecessors. These teeth have complex existing restorative work and exposed surfaces at risk to new and secondary caries as changes in saliva, dexterity and medication all combine to increase caries risk in individuals to varying extents.

In many countries, over a number of decades, there has been a failure to implement comprehensive caries prevention into mainstream general practice. The gap between what is taught in dental schools in clinical cariology and what is carried out and funded remains wide. At the same time the World Health Organization (WHO) and the World Health Assembly are giving advice to governments to re-orientate policies towards health promotion and prevention [4]. In framing policies and strategies for oral health, countries are being advised that 'particular emphasis should be laid on the following elements… Building of capacity *in oral-health systems oriented to disease prevention and primary health care,* oral-health services should be set up, *ranging from prevention, early diagnosis and intervention to provision of treatment and rehabilitation, and the management of oral health problems* of the population according to needs and to resources available' [4]. The resolution of the Sixtieth World Health Assembly – Oral health: action plan for promotion and integrated disease prevention – urges member states to adopt a number of 'measures to ensure that oral health is incorporated as appropriate into policies for the integrated prevention and treatment of chronic non-communicable and communicable diseases'. The other actions include recognition of the need 'to strengthen oral-health research and use evidence-based oral-health promotion and disease prevention in order to consolidate and adapt oral-health programmes, and to encourage the intercountry exchange of reliable knowledge and experience' [4].

The Purpose of this Book

The purpose of this book is to provide an up-to-date synthesis of the fields around the *detection, assessment, diagnosis and monitoring of caries* in which the available evidence is reviewed and current international views on best practice are summarized on how the information collected can be collated and synthesized to inform the planning, delivery and clinical evaluation of *patient-centred, comprehensive caries management.*

The evidence-based dentistry philosophy guides us to plan care that results in *doing the right thing, done right, at the right time for the right person.* This is why there is an increasing focus on patient-centred, personalized treatment plans, rather than a mechanistic focus, in which very different patients with different states of disease activity and different behaviours and needs end up with very similar 'automatic' care plans.

Treatment plans are now more *comprehensive* than was typically the case some decades ago, as clinicians (and patients) focus on more holistic and long-term plans. These treatment plans are not just about restoring individual teeth and not just about dental caries, they look at the needs and preferences of individuals. Dentists now have many more facets of information that it can be useful to collate and more treatment options available to them. The public health moves advocating changes towards the shared planning of care with patients links well with patient/customer-centred dental practices wanting to be commercially successful and to have satisfied, motivated and loyal patients return to the practice over an extended period.

The target audience for this book comprises those with an interest in dental caries and its clinical management; this should in no way detract from the parallel missions in the domains of dental public health, research or education.

The Role of the International Caries Detection and Assessment System

The aims and treatment elements referred to above all link with aspects of the International Caries Detection and Assessment System (ICDAS) and its framework. There is no exclusive relationship, the individual elements outlined in this book can and do stand alone. However, the authors wish to share the potential of the ICDAS methodology to enhance and enable the processes for the *detection, assessment, diagnosis and monitoring of caries* as well as for planning *patient-centred, comprehensive caries management.* The readers should make their assessment of the utility of the various criteria and tools outlined.

The shared vision for the ICDAS is that:
- it is a clinical visual caries scoring system for use in clinical practice, dental education, research and epidemiology;

- it is designed to lead to better-quality information to inform decisions about appropriate diagnosis, prognosis and clinical management at both the individual and public health levels;
- it provides a framework to support and enable personalized comprehensive caries management for improved long-term health outcomes.

The ICDAS came about as a collaborative, open, system following a number of initiatives seeking to better understand and improve caries 'diagnosis' and clinical management in an increasingly 'evidence-based' environment. There had been a number of attempts in the cariology community to better manage caries pathology, caries diagnosis and introduce more logical clinical management [5]. In 2001 in the USA, the National Institutes of Health convened a consensus development conference on the 'Diagnosis and management of dental caries throughout life' [6]. This international event considered a series of systematic and narrative reviews of the evidence on, amongst other topics, clinical applications and outcomes of using indicators of risk in caries management [7]. At the same time the caries research community was also reviewing methodology, evidence and consensus around caries detection and assessment in clinical trials [8] and looked at a review of visual and visuotactile detection of dental caries [9] and modern concepts of caries measurement [10].

These developments led to an international volunteer group meeting on a series of occasions to build on these initiatives to form the ICDAS Committee. This work led the group to submerge a number of discrete individual systems they were using into a common system incorporating the best of what was available and what was already in the literature in order to develop an international system for caries detection and assessment 'to facilitate caries epidemiology, research and appropriate clinical management' [11]. This system has continued to evolve and has been trialled in a number of settings [12]. In addition to the clinical visual focus on lesion detection and activity, the system has been designed to work with the outputs from diagnostic tools for early caries detection [13]. The ICDAS has been established as a charitable, not-for-profit foundation, in order to try and support the shared ICDAS vision outlined above. Details of its work and publications can be found on the worldwide web at www.icdas.org/.

The Move towards a More Preventive Focus in Clinical Caries Management

The trends in clinical caries management in recent decades have been around more clearly discriminating between those lesions, in specific patients, that would typically have *preventive care advised* as opposed to those lesions where, on the basis of synthesized information, *operative care* would be *advised* [14]. In the latter case, operative intervention is only planned when specific thresholds have been exceeded and preventive care is also provided to try to deal with the causative factors, rather than just the consequences of the disease. There has been a gradual international shift towards such an approach to minimal intervention dentistry [15], which has been supported by the Fédération Dentaire Internationale. Although the rates at which dentists in different countries have moved to embrace such a concept has been very variable [16], this now seems to be increasing globally. There are still gaps between current practice and international recommendations, and a blend of education and service development issues are needed to maintain progress and support some clinicians through a period of change.

The focus is also around showing how the appropriate use of clinical visual caries detection and assessment methods, combined with additional information on lesion detection and lesion activity, as well as synthesized information about the individual patient, can enable improved health care plans and outcomes in clinical cariology. There has been an increasing consensus that although there is a lack of high-quality randomized trials directly addressing the issues in routine clinical practice, at the individual patient level there should be an increasing recognition of the importance of caries risk status and personalized recall intervals [17, 18].

In addition to the activities within the ICDAS Committee, over recent years there has been a wealth of parallel activities and developments taken forward by individuals working within organizations such as the European Organization for Caries Research, the International Association for Dental Research Cariology Group, the Caries Management by Risk Assessment Groups, the American Dental Association, the Fédération Dentaire Internationale, the American Dental Education Association Cariology Special Interest Group and the Scottish Dental Clinical Effectiveness Programme (SDCEP). Contributions from these individuals and groups are made in the subsequent chapters and are gratefully acknowledged.

One key challenge in this area is the conflicting use of seemingly similar but different terms in the description of caries, caries (carious) lesions and how they are characterized. This is particularly marked as one travels between the domains of clinical practice, dental education, research and epidemiology, and the confusion produced serves as a barrier to communication and advancing clinical care.

The book includes a consensus glossary of terminology developed with a number of key stakeholders as it is vitally important that all concerned with caries and its management are clear about what is meant by different stages of the caries process and understand the specific meanings attached to the terms: detection; assessment; diagnosis; monitoring.

Figure 1 shows an updated version of an earlier caries cube [10], outlining 3 different types of caries measurement. It relates the *detection of lesion extent* on the front face (classifying different stages of disease severity with ICDAS codes), the *assessment of lesion activity* on the top face (making a snapshot assessment at a single examination) and *monitoring of lesion behaviour over time* on the side face (where the status of lesions is monitored over a series of time points using appropriate ICDAS codes).

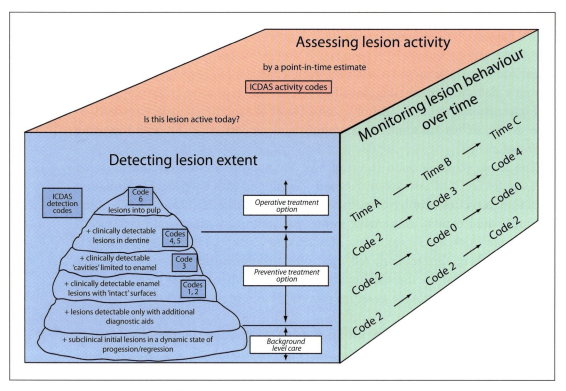

Fig. 1. The caries cube: relating the detection of lesion extent, assessment of lesion activity and monitoring of lesion behaviour over time.

It is important to understand the different clinical uses of these 3 types of caries measurement, all of which contribute to planning and assessing personalized caries management.

The ICDAS-enabled framework for patient-centred caries management has been used as the backbone structure for this volume. It outlines the information needs and the information flow required. Figure 2 comprises a graphic outlining the clinical framework. The ways in which the information is collected are outlined in the respective chapters which align to the framework. The chapter on personalized treatment planning [this vol., pp. 128–143] considers in more depth how the information is synthesized.

Chapter authors have been selected for their expertise in the various elements of cariology that the book and framework address. In some cases multiple authors have been selected to blend international evidence, practice and views in developing areas. For key chapters where the ICDAS Committee has built a consensus over an extended period, lead authors have written on behalf of the Committee.

The individual chapters of this volume are:

Clinical visual lesion detection (for the ICDAS Committee)
Traditional lesion detection aids
Novel lesion detection aids
Lesion activity assessment (for the ICDAS Committee)
Patient caries risk assessment
Dentition and lesion history
Assessing patient's health behaviours
Personalized treatment planning (for the ICDAS Committee)
Background level care
Traditional preventive treatment options
Novel preventive treatment options
Traditional operative treatment options
Novel operative treatment options
Recall, reassessment and monitoring
Implementation: improving caries detection, assessment, diagnosis and monitoring
Glossary of key terms (produced in collaboration with the ICDAS, European Organization for Caries Research and American Dental Education Association Cariology Special Interest Group – Caries Glossary Groups)

Where possible the chapters employ a consistent use of the key caries terminology as defined in the chapter by Longbottom et al. [this vol., pp. 209–216], based upon the work undertaken by the various groups to harmonize terminology in this area. The groups plan to continue the development of the glossary further. Given the differing needs and background of various 'users', and specifically groups as different as researchers (needing precision) and practitioners (needing simpler clarity), the glossary will be split into the 4 domains with levels of detail appropriate for clinical practice, dental education, caries research and caries epidemiology.

Where possible, chapters have included an estimation of the level of evidence that currently supports work in the field (see below), a list of research priorities (based on the gaps in the evidence base) as well as a list of implementation priorities (for getting research findings into practice).

Grading of Recommendations

The grading of recommendations for clinical practice on the basis of the strength of evidence reviewed is a complex and developing field. There are varieties of systems described and in place to do this, and all have been considered. It is a complex task to link the strength of evidence pertaining to a specific clinical intervention (as determined by the quality of the research available in the literature, including consideration of the study design and rigour) with a recommendation to use the intervention

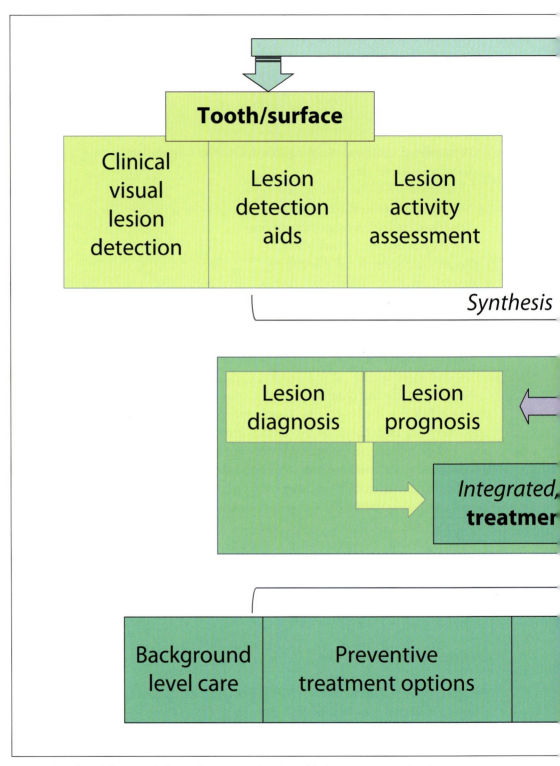

Fig. 2. The clinical framework for implementing ICDAS-enabled, patient-centred caries management.

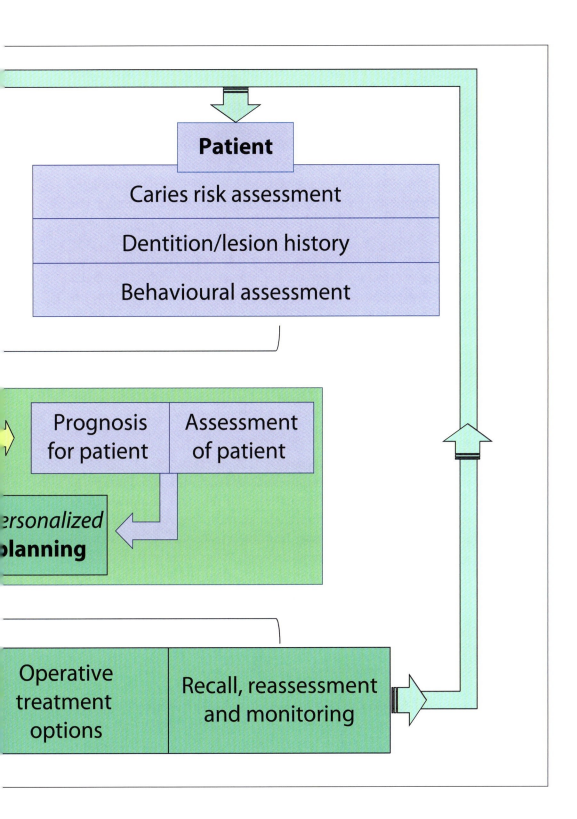

Introduction

for an individual patient. This challenge is greater still in cases where randomized controlled trial methodology is difficult or inappropriate and where evidence for new treatments is limited but is superior to current practice.

Having considered the available options, for this volume we have used, where appropriate, the system developed by the SDCEP. One of the major concerns that the SDCEP had with the existing systems was that there were occasions where the guidance development groups wished to highlight recommendations where there were existing legal professional regulatory requirements which were therefore considered to be mandatory (as in radiation protection and prevention of cross-infection). It was also considered that there was a number of areas where there was a general consensus regarding good professional practice yet there was no (or there was unlikely to be any) supporting evidence (in the foreseeable future). To incorporate these two situations into the grading system, a modified version of the GRADE system was developed using the SIGN (www.sign.ac.uk) levels of evidence (table 1). This scheme has been in place for the production of the first 3 guidance documents produced by the SDCEP and is being kept under review. In the chapters concerned, the recommendations are coded as R_m, R_s, R_w or R_e corresponding to the categories set out in table 1. In cariology there will be few recommendations which are legally considered as mandatory (R_m).

Other Applications of the ICDAS

The ICDAS aims to enhance the detection, assessment, diagnosis and monitoring of caries. As has been stated above, the target audience for this book comprises those with an interest in dental caries and its clinical management. It is vital to realize that this clinical focus should in no way detract from the parallel ICDAS missions (to lead to better-quality information to inform decisions about appropriate diagnosis, prognosis and clinical management at both the individual and public health levels) in the domains of dental public health/epidemiology, clinical research or dental education.

Dental Public Health/Epidemiology Example of the ICDAS

The ICDAS detection codes can and have been employed in epidemiological surveys of caries prevalence and health surveillance [19]. Figure 3 shows the 'Pitts adaptation' of the so-called WHO 'stepwise' approach to surveillance of non-communicable diseases for use with oral health indicators and the ICDAS options that this offers for use in dental public health/epidemiology.

In this approach step 1 addresses *questionnaire data* ('core' concerns pain, 'enhanced' is for oral health impact, and 'supplements' include estimates of quality of

Table 1. SDCEP grading scheme for recommendations

Symbol	Basis for recommendation
R_m	These recommendations are legal or professional regulatory requirements and are therefore considered to be **mandatory**
R_s	These recommendations are supported by **strong** evidence with limited bias (level 1++/1+/2++/2+)[1]
R_w	These recommendations are supported by **weak** evidence with some potential for bias (level 2+/3)[1]
R_e	These recommendations are based on a consensus of expert opinion (level 4)

[1] Referring to the SIGN evidence grading system (www.sign.ac.uk): level 2+ studies are regarded as strong evidence when the study designs are appropriate to address the question being considered. By contrast, level 2+ studies are regarded as weak evidence when they are not the most appropriate design, for example when addressing therapy questions

life), while step 2 comprises *physical measurements* of disease (which range from 'core', an ICDAS-approved modification for epidemiology in which air for drying is not available and cotton wool/gauze is used. In this case code 1 is combined with core 2 (as Code 1+2), and only codes 0 and 2–6 are used, to 'enhanced' where the full ICDAS codes 0–6 are used, to 'supplements' which is ICDAS + the use of caries detection aids). Step 3 is for *biochemical measurements* – as in cardiovascular disease (which is where future technology and caries activity assessments are expected to contribute to caries assessments in the future). It should be stressed that epidemiological data collected with ICDAS codes can also be computed to give backward-compatible D_3MF values in addition to the more complete ICDAS caries values.

Dental Education Example of the ICDAS

The ICDAS codes can and have been taught in dental education settings over the last few years. Examples include developments at the University of Indiana of caries risk forms and clinical management forms which have been in use for some time and where students are familiarized with the ICDAS codes, with the momentum achieved by the Caries Management by Risk Assessment (CAMBRA) groups and adoption of ICDAS by schools such as New York University. The teaching at the University of Copenhagen embraces the ICDAS for both dentists and hygienists, and in Scotland the teaching of the ICDAS is set to spread across all Scottish schools through the SDCEP process. In Australia minimally invasive dentistry has been taught for some years, and increasingly ICDAS codes are used [20].

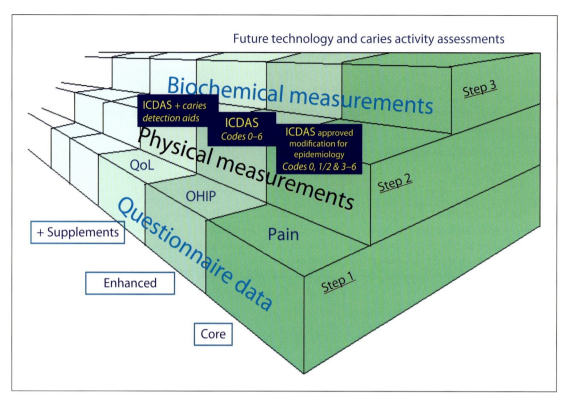

Fig. 3. Adaptation of the WHO 'stepwise' approach to surveillance of non-communicable diseases for use with oral health indicators and ICDAS options; shows ICDAS-approved modification where it is not feasible to record code 1s alone; data collected with the ICDAS can also be computed to give backward-compatible D_3MF values. OHIP = Oral health impact; QoL = quality of life.

Clinical Research Example of the ICDAS

The ICDAS has been very widely used in research settings over the last 7 years by different investigators in different countries and settings. The full range of peer-reviewed articles, abstracts and conference presentations can be accessed through updated lists on the ICDAS web page [21].

Acknowledgements

The author is extremely grateful to the following for assistance with this challenging task: the Karger Oral Science Coordinating Editors, for the invitation; Sandra Braun and the team at Karger for helping to make the book a reality; the ICDAS Committee, for their professional commitment to cariology and working to improve oral health by getting evidence into practice; the continuing leadership and partnership shown by ICDAS Co-Chair Amid Ismail and ICDAS Foundation

Co-Directors Kim Ekstrand and Dom Zero and their collaborators; Dr. Gail Toping, for her tireless coordination work with the ICDAS; the representatives working and sharing expertise on this publication from the European Organization for Caries Research, the International Association for Dental Research and the American Dental Education Association; Derek Richards, Jan Clarkson and the SDCEP for developing and sharing the grading system and an illustration; the staff of the Dental Health Services and Research Unit for their continuing support and in particular to Joyce Adams and Brian Bonner for their help with manuscripts; all supporters of the work of the ICDAS Foundation; Colgate – for their specific support via a no-strings educational grant, to enable the use of colour illustrations in this book.

References

1 Editorial – Oral Health: prevention is key. Lancet 2009;373:1.
2 Selwitz RH, Ismail AI, Pitts NB: Dental caries. Lancet 2007;369:51–59.
3 Elderton RJ: Clinical studies concerning re-restoration of teeth. Adv Dent Res 1990;4:4–9.
4 Petersen P-E: World Health Organization global policy for improvement of oral health – World Health Assembly 2007. Int Dent J 2008;58:115–121.
5 Ekstrand KR, Ricketts DN, Kidd EA: Occlusal caries: pathology, diagnosis and logical management. Dent Update 2001;28:380–387.
6 Diagnosis and management of dental caries throughout life: National Institutes of Health Consensus Development Conference statement, March 26–28, 2001. J Dent Educ 2001;65:935–1184.
7 Zero D, Fontana M, Lennon AM: Clinical applications and outcomes of using indicators of risk in caries management. J Dent Educ 2001;65:1132–1138.
8 Pitts NB, Stamm J: International Consensus Workshop on Caries Clinical Trials (ICW-CCT) final consensus statements: agreeing where the evidence leads. J Dent Res 2004;83(spec iss C):125–128.
9 Ismail AI: Visual and visuo-tactile detection of dental caries. J Dent Res 2004;83(spec iss C):56–66.
10 Pitts NB: Modern concepts of caries measurement. J Dent Res 2004;83(spec iss C):43–47.
11 Pitts NB: 'ICDAS' – an international system for caries detection and assessment being developed to facilitate caries epidemiology, research and appropriate clinical management. Community Dent Health 2004;21:193–198.
12 Ismail AI, Sohn W, Tellez M, Amaya A, Sen A, Hasson H, Pitts NB: Reliability of the International Caries Detection and Assessment System (ICDAS): an integrated system for measuring dental caries. Community Dent Oral Epidemiol 2007;35:170–178.
13 Zandoná AF, Zero DT: Diagnostic tools for early caries detection. J Am Dent Assoc 2006;137:1675–1684.
14 Pitts NB, Longbottom C: Preventive care advised (PCA)/operative care advised (OCA) – categorising caries by the management option. Community Dent Oral Epidemiol 1995;23:55–59.
15 Tyas MJ, Anusavice KJ, Frencken JE, Mount GJ: Minimal intervention dentistry – a review. FDI commission project 1-97. Int Dent J 2000;50:1–12.
16 Pitts NB: Are we ready to move from operative to non-operative/preventive treatment of dental caries in clinical practice? Caries Res 2004;38:294–304.
17 National Collaborating Centre for Acute Care, National Institute for Clinical Excellence (NICE): Dental Recall – Recall Interval between Routine Dental Examinations: Methods, Evidence and Guidance. London, Royal College of Surgeons of England, 2004, p 118. www.nice.org.uk/CG019full guideline.
18 Young DA, Featherstone JB, Roth JR: Caries management by risk assessment – a practitioner's guide. CDA J 2007;35:679–680.
19 Bourgeois DM, Christensen LB, Ottolenghi L, Llodra JC, Pitts NB, Senakola E (eds): Health Surveillance in Europe – European Global Oral Health Indicators Development Project Oral Health Interviews and Clinical Surveys: Guidelines. Lyon, Lyon I University Press, 2008.

20 Evans RW, Pakdaman A, Dennison PJ, Howe ELC: The Caries Management System: an evidence-based preventive strategy for dental practitioners – application for adults. Aust Dent J 2008;53:83–92.

21 International Caries Detection and Assessment System (ICDAS). www.icdas.org/.

N.B. Pitts
Dental Health Services and Research Unit, University of Dundee
Mackenzie Building, Kirsty Semple Way
Dundee DD2 4BF (UK)
Tel. +44 1382 420067, Fax +44 1382 420051, E-Mail n.b.pitts@cpse.dundee.ac.uk

Clinical Visual Caries Detection

G.V.A. Topping · N.B. Pitts, for the International Caries Detection and Assessment System Committee

Dental Health Services and Research Unit, University of Dundee, Dundee, UK

Abstract

The reliable and reproducible detection of dental caries by clinical examination has been recognized as a problem for decades with very variable approaches being taken to recognize and stage lesions along the continuum of caries – from very small initial lesions, just visible to the human eye, through more established white- and brown-spot lesions, to shadowing beneath the enamel and different extents of cavitation. Clinical caries lesion detection implies some objective method of determining whether or not disease is present, and many systems have been developed to improve the objectivity of examiners. The existence of a large number of different systems, using different definitions of caries detection thresholds, lesion staging and examination conditions has led to problems in comparing between studies and communicating across different dental domains. The International Caries Detection and Assessment System (ICDAS) has been developed from the best elements of previously published systems and is based upon the most robust evidence currently available to address the incompatibility of the systems currently used across the full breadth of cariology. The inherently visual ICDAS lesion detection codes are outlined for use with primary coronal caries, caries adjacent to restorations and sealants and for root surface caries. The ICDAS detection codes for primary coronal caries have been demonstrated to have the capability to record both enamel and dentinal caries in a reliable, valid and reproducible manner in both permanent and deciduous teeth and are being adopted increasingly in the domains of research, epidemiology, clinical practice and education.

Copyright © 2009 S. Karger AG, Basel

Clinical Visual Caries Detection Systems

The systematic recording of dental caries has been a focus of research and epidemiology for well in excess of half a century. In 1951, Backer-Dirks et al. [1] opened their publication with the remark 'The great stumbling block in scientific caries research is the difficulty of an exact estimation of caries incidence', and this remains a significant problem today. They also pointed out that it was very necessary to develop a method of reproducibly recording 'caries incipiens' for the exact evaluation of therapeutic measures to prevent caries. The search for such methods has resulted in the development of numerous systems for recording the presence or absence of caries at different thresholds of detection. Since at least 1966 there have been systems in use which included codes for non-cavitated lesions [2], this having been advocated more than 20 years earlier by Sognnaes [3]. Some of the most widely adopted systems however, such as those produced for 'Basic Methods' by the World Health Organization (WHO) and Radike [4], have provision to record caries only at the dentinal threshold of detection – the WHO, who used in the 1970s to have systems including enamel caries, has in recent decades only published 'basic methods' for surveys which have been at the dentinal level and included dentinal lesions without frank cavitation to the count of decay experience only towards the start of this millennium [5, 6].

The effects of varying detection thresholds on the prevalence of disease detected was demonstrated by Pitts and Fyffe [7] who showed using data from Hong Kong collected in the 1980s that, although criteria from different surveys might be interpreted as being similar, slight changes in the detection threshold of examinations on the same group of individuals led to large differences in their reported caries prevalence. This illustrated the need for harmonization of at least the interpretation of caries thresholds. Further epidemiological work conducted by Ismail and co-workers in Canada has also demonstrated the significant proportion of caries which is ignored in selecting a detection threshold which excludes lesions which are not cavitated [8].

Even in the past two decades there have been many proposals for systems which take these points into account and which include proposals for grading both early and established dental caries [8–10]. Furthermore, in the recognition that detecting caries alone is of limited use without assessing its activity, a number of systems have been developed which attempt to record both lesion presence and activity [9, 11, 12]. The importance of assessing lesion activity is also fundamental to clinical decision-making and those in this field of research such as Nyvad et al. [11–13], as well as a number of the International Caries Detection and Assessment System (ICDAS) Committee members, have progressed this area significantly in recent years. Further discussion of the importance of the assessment of caries activity and the current research in this area can be found in the relevant chapter of this monograph [pp. 52–62].

Background of the International Caries Detection and Assessment System

There have been several conferences held during the last decade which have included debate on, or have focussed specifically on, caries detection and assessment. Examples include the 50th Anniversary European Organization for Caries Research Congress on Cariology in the 21st Century [13] and the series of published proceedings from the Indiana Conferences on Early Detection of Dental Caries [14–16]. One particular such meeting, which focussed upon the perspective of caries clinical trials but also considered the wider caries agenda, was held in 2002 [17].

This was supported by organizations such as the Fédération Dentaire Internationale, International Association for Dental Research and the major dentifrice companies. The 4-day meeting involved 95 participants from 23 countries with representatives from academia, industry, statisticians and regulators. This International Consensus Workshop on Caries Clinical Trials (ICW-CCT) worked towards international consensus on the future of caries clinical trials based upon research evidence in this field; systematic reviews were undertaken on key topic areas in order to summarize and interpret the research. The final consensus statements [17] included the following:

- There is some confusion with the terminology employed in the literature around *caries diagnosis* (which should imply a human professional summation of all available data), *lesion detection* (which implies some objective method of determining whether or not disease is present) and *lesion assessment* (which aims to characterize or monitor a lesion, once it has been detected)
- The understanding of the caries process has progressed far beyond the point of restricting the evidence for dental caries to the D_2 (caries in enamel only) or D_3 (caries in enamel and dentine) levels of cavitation
- For future clinical trials, recording only cavitated lesions as an outcome measure is becoming outmoded
- The workshop participants also recommended that 'in light of the evidence reviewed, both here and elsewhere, pertaining to modern caries definitions and measurement concepts, the participants supported a statement recommending that in future controlled clinical trials, caries measurement methods are employed which: (1) are capable of accurately capturing at any given point in time the manifestations of the caries process in dental hard tissues (enamel and dentine); (2) when applied sequentially, can monitor definitive changes in manifestations of the caries process over time, over and above any background "noise" from normal levels of de- and remineralization, or from variations attributable to the caries detection system(s) employed; (3) when applied sequentially, can differentiate actual product effects in terms of group differences in lesion initiation and lesion behaviour (progression, arrest and/or regression)'

Across the fields of clinical research and epidemiology, there have been many systems developed which address some, but not all, of the concerns of the ICW-CCT workshop. The large number of systems in use at that point in time is testament to the fact that it is hard to categorize a complex disease like dental caries into a scale because the process is continuous, and determining between different stages of the disease can be subjective.

One of the systematic reviews undertaken for the ICW-CCT meeting by Ismail [18] was on the topic of visual and visuotactile detection of dental caries. The review found that the majority of then current caries detection systems were ambiguous and did not measure the disease process at different stages. It also noted that while newer caries detection criteria measured different stages of the caries process, there were inconsistencies in how the caries process was measured. The review concluded that there was an urgent need to address the answers to the following questions:

1. What stage of the caries process should be measured?
2. What are the definitions for each selected stage?
3. What is the best clinical approach to detect each stage on different tooth surfaces?
4. What protocols of examiners' training can provide the highest degree of examiner reliability?

The challenges posed by the ICW-CCT workshop, Ismail's systematic review of the literature and other sources of evidence in this area [10, 19–23] led an ad hoc group to start the development of the ICDAS.

The initial goal of that committee was to develop an integrated clinical detection and assessment system of dental caries for research and clinical practice, with the capability of visually recording both enamel and dentinal caries and address the incompatibility of the terminology, criteria and grading systems currently used across the partially overlapping fields of caries epidemiology, clinical caries research and clinical caries management.

The first meeting of the ICDAS core group, co-chaired by Prof. Nigel Pitts and Prof. Amid Ismail took place in Dundee, Scotland, in April 2002. By early 2003, the group had collated current evidence relating to the detection of dental caries and had reviewed all of the previously published systems for caries detection and assessment. Pulling the best evidence from all of the previously published systems together along with additional research contributing to our current understanding of cariology, a proposal was developed for the 'ICDAS I' of recording dental caries. In March 2003, an expert group of 65 cariologists from around the world were brought together by the ICDAS core group in Baltimore to challenge and improve the proposed criteria. The resulting 'ICDAS II' criteria have been in use since then, and there have been 11 formal ICDAS workshops in Europe, North and South America which have involved researchers from all around the world. The workshops have shared research agendas and findings and have sought to facilitate the development and implementation of an 'open' system which provides a 'wardrobe' of validated criteria to use for caries detection and assessment. A charitable ICDAS Foundation has been set up to carry forward the shared ICDAS Vision outlining its purpose.

- The ICDAS is a clinical visual scoring system for use in dental education, clinical practice, research and epidemiology
- The ICDAS is designed to lead to better-quality information to inform decisions about appropriate diagnosis, prognosis and clinical management at both the individual and public health levels
- The ICDAS provides a framework to support and enable personalized comprehensive caries management for improved long-term health outcomes

Application of the International Caries Detection and Assessment System

The ICDAS was developed to be applicable in a number of different realms internationally (fig. 1); as already stated, it is based upon the best evidence from clinical research and applies not only to this field, but also to epidemiology and clinical practice. Furthermore, it is a valuable tool for the communication of modern concepts of cariology in both undergraduate and postgraduate dental education. An educational software package has been developed in partnership with the full ICDAS Committee to assist in the educating of students and clinicians in the use of the ICDAS [24].

The ICDAS was developed to provide a system for caries detection that would allow for comparison of data collected not only in these different realms, but also in different locations as well as at different points of time. The ICDAS was also developed to bring forward the current understanding of the process of initiation and progression of dental caries to the fields of epidemiological and clinical research. The coordinating committee also took into consideration developing a system that has wider utility for dental practitioners. If dental caries is classified using agreed upon criteria and systems, then comparison of findings by researchers, epidemiologists and clinicians from different countries would be feasible. It must be recognized that clinical visual lesion detection provides the foundation information for caries assessment and care planning. It should be further appreciated that many other facets of information, outlined in the following chapters, are also required to make the decisions required to deliver patient-centred, comprehensive caries management.

Some Examples of the Use of International Caries Detection and Assessment System Lesion Detection in Different Fields

Clinical Practice
From the very beginning, the ICDAS was designed not just as a tool for researchers and epidemiologists, but also for use in clinical practice. The ICDAS caries detection codes on their own cannot provide all the information needed for planning the appropriate management of caries; however, these simple codes are not only a common language for the communication of findings from the fields of research and epidemiology, but also have other valuable applications to clinical practice. Firstly, detailed recording of caries status should be part of every patient's initial oral assessment to allow for comparison over time, and the ICDAS codes allow a 7-point staging of caries to be recorded. Using these codes, a clinician can see over time whether preventive measures are being effective or not for their patients. The assessment of caries lesions and risk assessment of patients are topics in other chapters of this book. Secondly, it has been found by clinicians using the ICDAS codes that these are an excellent method of communicating with patients about their dental health and their success or otherwise in managing lesions which have been detected and in preventing

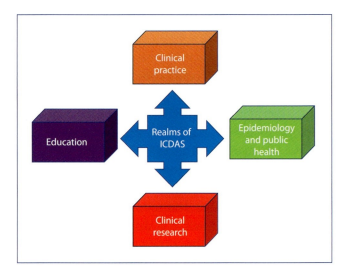

Fig. 1. Application of ICDAS across different areas of dentistry.

new lesions. The ICDAS has been included within the Scottish draft Dental Clinical Effectiveness Programme Guidance currently proposed for use in clinical practice for the comprehensive oral assessment of patients in Scotland.

Clinical Research

In the field of clinical research there are numerous examples of both research into the ICDAS and research using it. There are too many of such to list here but there have been in excess of 22 journal publications, 3 book chapters and more than 50 presentations on the subject of ICDAS at scientific and professional meetings in a range of countries. Further information on the ICDAS in the literature can be found on the website ICDAS.org where an up-to-date list is maintained. The focus of research into the ICDAS over the past few years has been to complete the gaps in the areas where existing evidence was weak and to test the system for validity, reliability and reproducibility. The research in this area is further summarized in the following sections:

Education

The ICDAS also has a clear role within dental education, both at the undergraduate and postgraduate level. Since the system is based upon the most recent and most robust evidence available on cariology, it is a valuable resource for discussing modern cariology and for putting this knowledge into practice in the dental clinic. Since the ICDAS includes the staging of caries from its earliest visual signs, it is a useful tool for introducing the concept of caries prevention and monitoring and again is a useful tool for communication between staff and students about the disease. It is hoped that the ICDAS can help to promote the conservation of the dental hard tissues where possible and the appropriate use of preventive therapies and minimal intervention. Again this is the focus of other chapters within this book. There is currently a great deal of interest from dental educational establishments all around the world to include the ICDAS within the dental curriculum; this includes schools in Europe, North and South America. An innovative teaching resource has been produced for those with an interest in the ICDAS, and this is in the form of an e-learning package. The ICDAS protocols for caries detection and the ICDAS criteria are presented in interactive modules which have an element of testing to promote standardization of the use of the ICDAS codes.

Epidemiology
The ICDAS has been embraced in a number of epidemiological settings. Two large-scale examples include a survey of 6-, 12- and 15-year-old children's dental health in Iceland in 2005, which in addition to using the ICDAS also took bitewing radiographs of the children [25], and the European Global Oral Health Indicators Development Programme [26]. The ICDAS was selected as the preferred measure for recording dental caries severity by a panel of European experts tasked with choosing essential oral health indicators for the whole of Europe in an effort to harmonize and compare information from all of the member states. Caries severity was just one of the 15 clinical indicators chosen. A pilot project to assess the feasibility of collecting this harmonized information was carried out in 2008 in 10 countries across Europe. An interesting feature of this project is the use of 'sentinel dentists', regular general practitioners, to collect the epidemiological information in dental practice. For this project ICDAS examinations were conducted by 146 dentists on nearly 3,000 patients, and regarding the ICDAS the pilot study concluded that there were no major problems in its use or acceptability.

Examination Conditions

To understand the measurement of caries, it is important to review basic concepts. Sound enamel is translucent and microporous. After repeated episodes of demineralization exceeding remineralization, the subsurface enamel increases in microporosity. This leads to a change in the refractive index of enamel and hence its optical properties. The first sign of carious change is a change in translucency and light refraction of enamel which is seen only when the surface is dehydrated for a short period. If demineralization continues and mineral loss increases, further reduction occurs in the refractive index of enamel which means that such lesions can now be seen without the need to dehydrate the surface of the lesion – these lesions are seen even when the surface is covered with saliva and represent a more advanced stage of dental caries than those which can only be seen after air-drying. This property of demineralized enamel leads to one of the primary requirements for applying the full ICDAS and that is availability of compressed air to reveal the earliest visual signs of caries.

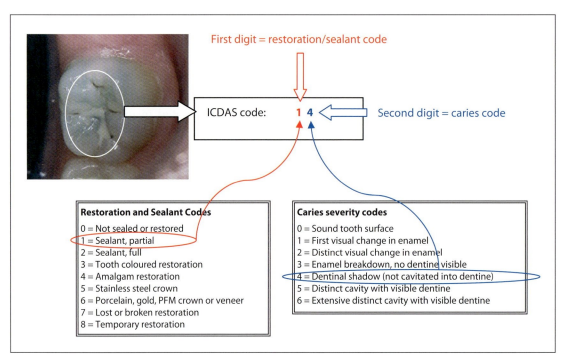

Fig. 2. ICDAS coding for restoration status and caries severity. PFM = Porcelain fused to metal.

Another fundamental condition for the detection of enamel caries in particular is the removal of plaque from the tooth surfaces prior to examination. Since caries forms in areas of plaque stagnation and would therefore remain hidden from sight, this is a very important part of the ICDAS examination. It is highly advisable that the teeth are cleaned with a toothbrush or a prophylaxis head/cup before the examination, and it is recommended that the approximal surfaces of teeth are also flossed to remove retentive plaque.

The ICDAS examination is almost purely visual but can be aided by a ball-ended explorer in order to remove any remaining plaque and debris, to lightly check for surface contour and minor cavitation and to confirm the presence of tooth-coloured restorations and sealants. The use of a sharp explorer is not necessary because it does not add to accuracy of the detection and may damage the enamel surface covering early carious lesions [27, 28].

Examining for Caries Outside a Dental Office/Clinic

Ideal examination conditions are not always possible outside the dental surgery setting. In recognition of this a very basic ICDAS examination may be conducted

Table 1. ICDAS codes for restoration status

Code	Description
0	Unrestored and unsealed
1	Partial sealant – a sealant which does not cover all pits and fissures of the tooth surface
2	Full sealant
3	Tooth-coloured restoration
4	Amalgam restoration
5	Stainless-steel crown
6	Porcelain, gold or preformed metal crown or veneer
7	Lost or broken restoration
8	Temporary restoration

without the aid of compressed air for dehydrating lesions. ICDAS coding undertaken in these less ideal circumstances will mean that the earliest signs of caries will be missed and therefore the threshold of the examination is altered. It is important that those reporting on surveys or studies in these conditions state this clearly as it will affect comparison with other studies. It is also important that no compromise is made with regard to the teeth being clean prior to inspection; this is an essential condition for any ICDAS examination.

Two Stages of ICDAS Coding

Recording the status of dental caries using the ICDAS is a 2-stage process. Figure 2 illustrates how the 2-digit code is composed of a code for the restorative status of the surface followed by a code for the caries severity.

The first stage is to classify each tooth surface on its restoration status. The criteria differentiate between partially and fully sealed tooth surfaces and between different restorative materials. These codes are the first of 2 digits coding the status of each tooth surface. The codes are listed in table 1.

International Caries Detection and Assessment System Severity Codes

The second digit of the ICDAS criteria records the caries severity of a tooth surface. Since clinically we rely on visual signs (change in colour, cavitation) which represent manifestations of a relatively advanced caries process, the ICDAS criteria incorporate concepts from the research conducted by Ekstrand et al. [20, 29] and other caries detection systems described in the systematic review conducted by Ismail [18], which indicates that measurement of non-cavitated carious lesions in enamel or dentine can be based on visual topography at the surface level. While such systems are not perfectly accurate, they have both content and correlational validity with histological depth of carious lesions. The ICDAS measures the surface changes and potential histological depth of carious lesions by relying on surface characteristics.

Ekstrand et al. [29] correlated the severity of carious lesions and their histological depth. White-spot lesions, which require air-drying, are most likely to be limited to the outer half of the enamel. The depth of a white- or brown-spot lesion which is obvious without air-drying is located some place between the inner half of the enamel and the outer third of the dentine. Localized enamel breakdown due to caries, with no visible dentine, indicates that the lesion extends to the middle third of the dentine. In addition, a greyish, brownish or bluish shadow of the dentine shining up through apparently intact enamel also indicates a lesion extending to the middle third of dentine. Frank cavities with visible dentine indicate that a lesion has been extended to the inner third of dentine. Further research confirming this relationship between the visual caries detection codes of the ICDAS and histological depth is reviewed further in this chapter. Figure 3 illustrates the relationship between ICDAS caries severity codes and the typical histological appearance of such lesions.

The ICDAS caries severity codes range from 0 (sound) to 6 (extensive distinct cavity exposing dentine) relating the visual signs of caries with their depth into the tooth surface (fig. 4). The full description of these codes can be found in the ICDAS II criteria document available on the ICDAS Foundation website ICDAS.org. The following descriptions summarize the caries severity codes.

Sound Tooth Surface: Code 0

There should be no evidence of caries (no change, or only questionable change, in enamel translucency after prolonged air-drying, with a suggested drying time of 5 s). Surfaces with developmental defects such as enamel hypoplasias, fluorosis, tooth wear (attrition, abrasion and erosion), and extrinsic or intrinsic stains should be recorded as sound. Examiners should also score as sound a surface with multiple stained fissures if this is seen in other pits and fissures, a presentation which is consistent with staining from dietary sources rather than caries. Staining seen around restoration margins that are not associated with other signs of caries should be coded 0 as well as non-carious marginal defects of less than 0.5 mm in the absence of signs of caries (fig. 5 b, c).

First Visual Change in Enamel: Code 1

Code 1 lesions represent the earliest signs of dental caries which can be detected visually. The level of demineralization of these lesions is such that, if the moisture

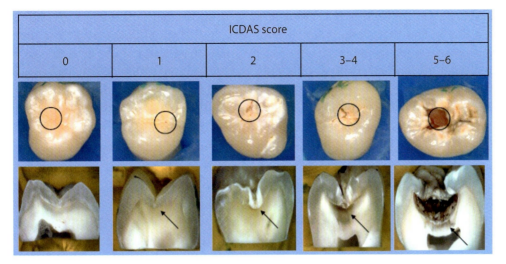

Fig. 3. ICDAS codes and histology. Images provided by courtesy of Dr. A. Ferreira Zandona, University of Indiana.

0		Sound tooth surface
1		First visual change in enamel
2		Distinct visual change in enamel
3		Localised enamel breakdown due to caries with no visible dentine
4		Underlying dark shadow from dentine (with or without enamel breakdown)
5		Distinct cavity with visible dentine
6		Extensive distinct cavity with visible dentine

Fig. 4. ICDAS codes for caries severity.

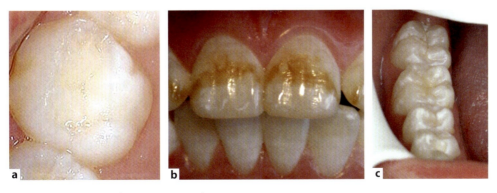

Fig. 5a–c. Examples of ICDAS caries code 0.

Clinical Visual Caries Detection

is removed from their surface with prolonged air-drying, their optical properties are altered and these lesions which were previously hard to distinguish from normal enamel when the tooth was wet become more opaque and can be detected. Such lesions in the pits and fissures can in time pick up staining which makes them easier to detect without air-drying, and therefore the ICDAS codes describe code 1 lesions separately for these two locations. These darkly discoloured lesions can look similar to tea- or coffee-stained pits and fissures (code 0). Such non-caries-related staining however tends to be seen in almost all pits and fissures symmetrically (fig. 6).

Code 1: Pits and Fissures
Some code 1 lesions in the pits and fissures show no evidence of any change in colour attributable to caries when viewed wet, but after prolonged air-drying (approx. 5 s is suggested to adequately dehydrate a carious lesion in enamel), a carious opacity of discolouration (brown or white lesions) becomes visible with an appearance which is not consistent with sound enamel. Other code 1 lesions, which have picked up staining from the oral environment, can be seen even when the tooth is wet. These lesions exhibit a change of colour because of caries which is not consistent with the clinical appearance of sound enamel. To be recorded as a code 1, these lesions must be confined to the base of the pit/fissure and may be seen when the tooth is wet or dry. The appearance of these lesions must be differentiated from the staining described in code 0 which is not attributable to caries.

Code 1: Smooth Surfaces
When seen wet there is no evidence of any change in colour attributable to carious activity, but after prolonged air-drying a carious opacity (which may be white or brown) is visible that is not consistent with the clinical appearance of sound enamel. On the approximal smooth surfaces, these can often only be viewed from the buccal or lingual/palatal directions.

Distinct Visual Change in Enamel: Code 2

If an enamel lesion loses further mineral, the optical properties alter once again. The demineralization of these later-stage enamel lesions is such that they become visible even when the tooth is viewed wet.

When wet, code 2 lesions exhibit either (i) carious opacity (white-spot lesion) and/or (ii) brown carious discolouration which is wider than the base of the natural fissure/fossa and has an appearance which is not consistent with the clinical appearance of sound enamel (these lesions can also be seen when the tooth surface is dried). Although air-drying is not necessary to detect code 2 lesions, it can be helpful to remove surface moisture to examine the surface of the enamel more clearly for signs of cavitation to distinguish between code 2 lesions which have (to the naked eye)

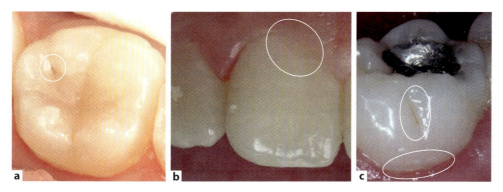

Fig. 6a–c. Examples of ICDAS caries code 1.

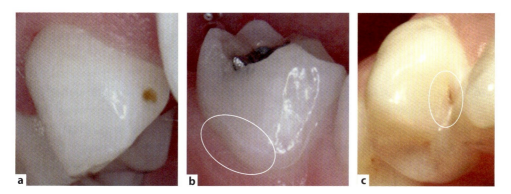

Fig. 7a–c. Examples of ICDAS caries code 2.

intact enamel surfaces (fig. 7) and code 3 lesions which have localized breakdown of the enamel.

Localized Enamel Breakdown because of Caries with No Visible Dentine or Underlying Shadow: Code 3

When caries has reached the stage that there has been so much loss of mineral from the enamel structure that it is grossly weakened, the enamel surface begins to break down and surface discontinuity can be visualized. Such lesions when viewed wet have a distinct carious opacity (white-spot lesion) and/or brown carious discolouration which is not consistent with the clinical appearance of sound enamel. In the pits and fissures, this is wider than the natural fissure/fossa – when dried for approximately 5 s a carious loss of tooth structure (opaque white, brown or dark brown walls) at the entrance to, or within, the pit or fissure/fossa can be visualized. The loss of enamel structure may be such that the fissure or fossa can appear substantially and unnaturally wider than normal; however, a code 3 lesion will not have exposed dentine in the walls or base of the cavity/discontinuity. If in doubt, or to confirm the visual assessment, a ball-ended probe can be used gently across a tooth surface to confirm the presence of a cavity apparently confined to enamel. This is achieved by sliding the ball end along the suspect surface and a limited discontinuity is detected if the ball drops into the surface of the enamel cavity/discontinuity. If any exposed dentine can be seen, this lesion should be coded as an ICDAS code 5.

In a restored tooth, a gap between a restoration and the tooth of less than 0.5 mm but associated with an opacity or discolouration consistent with demineralization should be coded 3 (fig. 8).

Underlying Dark Shadow from Dentine with or without Localized Enamel Breakdown (but without Cavitation into Dentine): Code 4

Code 4 lesions are histologically more advanced than code 3 lesions though there is some overlap between the depth of these two codes. Code 4 lesions appear as shadows of discoloured dentine visible through apparently intact enamel which may or may not exhibit localized breakdown (loss of continuity of the surface that is not exposing the dentine). The shadow appearance is often more noticeable when the surface is wet and may appear as grey, blue or brown. In a tooth restored with amalgam it can be difficult to distinguish the shine-through of the restoration from a carious shadow.

Code 4 is only recorded on surfaces where the caries originated. This is not usually a problem for examiners when the lesion originated on the occlusal surface but there can be confusion with large approximal lesions. In these instances the dentinal involvement of the cavity is often seen as shadowing through the occlusal surface even though the caries did not originate in the fissures of that surface. This is shown in figure 9b. The occlusal surface would not be coded as 4 because the lesion originated from the approximal surface. This is clearer in figure 10b where the approximal lesion can be directly visualized as a code 5, the shadowing related to undermined enamel from this lesion can be seen from the occlusal surface but should not be recorded to that surface as code 4 because the lesion did not originate here.

Distinct Cavity with Visible Dentine: Code 5

As caries progresses further, undermined enamel may eventually break down to expose dentine. A code 5 lesion is defined as being cavitation present due to caries in opaque or discoloured enamel exposing the dentine beneath. The tooth when viewed wet may have darkening of the dentine visible through the enamel. Once dried for 5

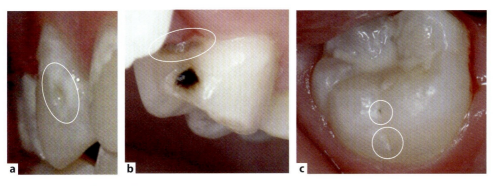

Fig. 8a–c. Examples of ICDAS caries code 3.

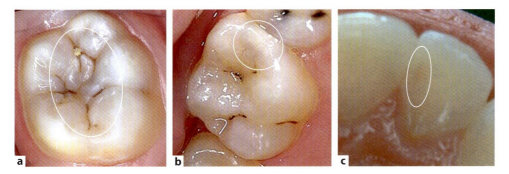

Fig. 9a–c. Examples of ICDAS caries code 4.

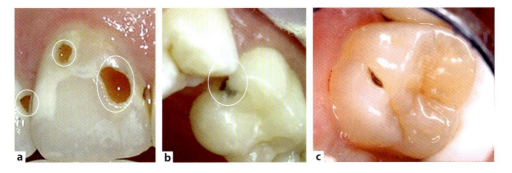

Fig. 10a–c. Examples of ICDAS caries code 5.

s there is visual evidence of loss of tooth structure – frank cavitation. In the pits and fissures there is visual evidence of demineralization [opaque (white), brown or dark brown walls] at the entrance to or within the pit or fissure, and dentine is exposed. Code 5 lesions involve less than half of the surface of the tooth.

A ball-ended probe can be used to confirm the presence of a cavity in dentine. This is achieved by sliding the ball end along the suspect surface and a dentine cavity

Clinical Visual Caries Detection 29

is detected if the ball enters the opening of the cavity and the base is into dentine. (In pits or fissures, the thickness of enamel is between 0.5 and 1.0 mm.) Please note that deep pulpal dentine should not be probed.

In a restored tooth, the gap between restoration and tooth should be larger than 0.5 mm to be coded as 5, and there will be dentine exposed in the gap.

Extensive Distinct Cavity with Visible Dentine (Involving Half of the Tooth Surface or More): Code 6

When at least half of the tooth surface is cavitated to expose dentine, the appropriate ICDAS code is 6. In these lesions there is obvious loss of tooth structure, the cavity is both deep and wide, and dentine is clearly visible on the walls and at the base of the cavity (fig. 11).

Caries Detection in Restored Teeth and on Roots

Caries Adjacent to Restorations and Sealants

Since carious lesions adjacent to restorations are thought to be analogous with primary caries, the broad principles applied to the criteria for primary caries are also applied to caries adjacent to restorations and sealants where relevant. However, it should be noted that the scientific basis for doing so has not been established, and the literature in the area of secondary caries is far more limited than for primary coronal caries. Much of the work which has been conducted has been done under 'ideal' conditions within the laboratory setting, and even then most have found poor correlations between visual signs and the histological findings.

Although caries associated with restorations is histologically similar to primary caries, its features cause certain diagnostic problems, including difficulties in the differentiation among restoration margin discrepancies (marginal integrity, discolouration of the tooth at restoration margin), secondary caries and residual caries [30].

Sharp probing for signs of secondary caries has all of the limitations and drawbacks associated with its use for primary caries detection. In addition, probing restored teeth can be misleading as a probe may become impacted in a margin discrepancy that is not in fact carious. It has been demonstrated that discolouration at the restoration margin is difficult to evaluate, as shown by a 'moderate' interexaminer agreement (κ = 0.49) [31]. In part this is due to the variety of causes of discolouration found next to amalgam in particular. It is not always predictive of secondary caries, as a large amalgam restoration or its corrosion products may discolour the tooth grey or blue without caries being present. It has also been suggested that slowly progressing lesions are darkly stained [32], probably from exogenous dietary sources such as tea or coffee. It

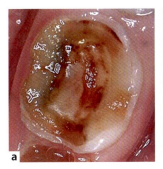 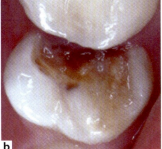 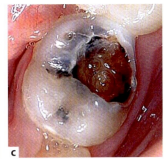

Fig. 11a–c. Examples of ICDAS caries code 6.

is possible that lesions that are most obvious clinically because of their colour may be the ones that are inactive, arrested or slowly progressing [33, 34]. Although corrosion products are known to form around amalgam fillings and are dark coloured, Kidd et al. [35] found similar levels of staining around amalgam fillings to that found around tooth-coloured restorations.

A number of studies have been conducted to investigate the association between shadowing or grey discolouration and the presence or absence of caries, some concluding that there is a statistically significant association [35–37] whilst others found no such relationship [38, 39].

In conclusion, therefore, it should be noted that whilst many studies have shown that grey discolouration or shadowing at the margins of restorations is statistically significantly associated with caries, recording this as non-cavitated dentinal caries is likely to result in an overestimation of the amount of disease. The confounding of shadowing due to restoration colour means that there are likely to be more false-positives than in unrestored teeth if discolouration or shadowing alone is used to predict the presence of caries.

The 2-digit recording system of the ICDAS allows users to record the restoration status of a tooth surface as well as the severity of carious lesions.

Root Caries

Root surface caries is similar to enamel caries, but unlike enamel caries, the surface can become softened and bacteria penetrate further into the tissue at an earlier stage of lesion development. A systematic review commissioned for the National Institutes of Health Consensus Development Conference on Dental Caries Diagnosis and Management throughout Life concluded that there is 'insufficient' evidence on the validity of clinical diagnostic systems for root caries [40]. However, the review only included clinical studies that used histology to validate the clinical caries diagnosis. This inclusion criterion excluded the vast majority of the literature on root caries.

Surveys describing the clinical appearance of root caries began to appear in the literature in the early 1970s, and many surveys and longitudinal studies on root caries were reported over the next two decades. Since the early 1990s, however, very few clinical studies on root caries have been conducted. These clinical studies primarily used diagnostic criteria proposed by several investigators [41–45].

Generally root caries lesions have been described as having a distinct outline and presenting with a discoloured appearance in relation to the surrounding non-carious root. Many root caries lesions are cavitated, although this is not necessarily the case with early lesions. The base of the cavitated area can be soft, leathery or hard to probing. Probing of root caries lesions with a sharp explorer using controlled, modest pressure may however create surface defects that prevent complete remineralization of the lesion [46]. Therefore, for detection and classification of root caries utilizing ICDAS criteria, examiners are directed to use a Community Periodontal Index probe [6].

Root caries is frequently observed near the cemento-enamel junction, although lesions can appear anywhere on the root surface. Lesions usually occur near (within 2 mm) the crest of the gingival margin. The distinction between an active and an arrested lesion further complicates clinical detection of root caries. The colour of root lesions has been used as an indication of lesion activity. Active lesions have been described as yellowish or light brown in colour whereas arrested lesions appear darkly stained. However, colour has subsequently been shown not to be a reliable indicator of caries activity [47, 48].

Since the clinical signs of lesions are considered to be different for active versus arrested root caries and the clinical signs associated with lesion activity have yet to be validated, the criteria proposed within the ICDAS incorporate all of the reported clinical signs, and therefore consider both lesion detection and assessment together unlike the criteria for coronal caries.

The presence of cavitation (loss of surface integrity) associated with a root caries lesion does not necessarily imply lesion activity. Non-cavitated (early) root caries lesions are almost universally considered to be active. However, a cavitated lesion may be either active or arrested. Lesion activity has been linked to lesion depth [49], but this clinical observation has not been verified.

The texture of a root caries lesion has also been linked to lesion activity. Active lesions have been described as soft or leathery compared to arrested lesions that have a hard texture. There is supporting laboratory evidence from a study that used microbiological indicators for lesion activity that 'soft' or 'leathery' lesions on root surfaces are more heavily infected with bacteria than are 'hard' root surfaces [48].

Root caries lesions that occur closely adjacent to (within 2 mm) the crest of the gingival crest are considered to be active whereas lesions that occur on the root surface more distant from the gingival crest are more likely to be arrested. There is microbiological evidence to support this clinical observation [50].

The determination of root caries activity is probably more closely related to decisions regarding treatment or management than to the determination of the presence of caries on the tooth root. Published reports on the clinical measurement of root caries were consulted in developing the ICDAS criteria [42, 43, 51, 52]. Given the paucity and generally low level of the scientific evidence, the ICDAS Coordinating Committee recommends that the following clinical criteria be used for the detection and classification of root caries:

1. colour (light/dark brown, black);
2. texture (smooth, rough);
3. appearance (shiny or glossy, matte or non-glossy);
4. perception on gentle probing (soft, leathery, hard);
5. cavitation (loss of anatomical contour).

Additionally, the outline of the lesion and its location on the root surface are useful in detecting root caries lesions. Root caries appears as a distinct, clearly demarcated circular or linear discolouration at the cemento-enamel junction or wholly on the root surface.

Codes for the Detection and Classification of Carious Lesions on the Root Surfaces

One score should be assigned per root surface. The facial, mesial, distal and lingual root surfaces of each tooth should be classified as follows.

Code E
If the root surface cannot be visualized directly as a result of gingival recession or by gentle air-drying, then it is excluded. Surfaces covered entirely by calculus can be excluded or, preferably, the calculus can be removed prior to determining the status of the surface. Removal of calculus is recommended for clinical trials and longitudinal studies.

Code 0
The root surface does not exhibit any unusual discolouration that distinguishes it from the surrounding or adjacent root areas nor does it exhibit a surface defect either at the cemento-enamel junction or wholly on the root surface. The root surface has a natural anatomical contour, *or* the root surface may exhibit a definite loss of surface continuity or anatomical contour that is not consistent with the dental caries process. This loss of surface integrity is usually associated with dietary influences or habits such as abrasion or erosion. These conditions usually occur on the facial surface. These areas are typically smooth, shiny and hard. Abrasion is characterized by a clearly defined outline with a sharp border, whereas erosion has a more diffuse border. Neither condition shows discolouration.

Code 1

There is a clearly demarcated area on the root surface or at the cemento-enamel junction that is discoloured (light/dark brown, black) but there is no cavitation (loss of anatomical contour <0.5 mm) present.

Code 2

There is a clearly demarcated area on the root surface or at the cemento-enamel junction that is discoloured (light/dark brown, black) and there is cavitation (loss of anatomical contour ≥0.5 mm) present.

ICDAS Reproducibility, Sensitivity and Specificity

During the development of the ICDAS criteria in August 2002, the 20 participants in the workshop examined the occlusal surfaces of 57 extracted teeth. The consensus of all participants was used to define the clinical status of the occlusal surfaces. The teeth were kept moist in containers and were sectioned and examined under a magnifying lens (×10). Each designated area was scored using the scale of Ricketts et al. [23] into:

0 = no enamel demineralization;

1 = enamel demineralization limited to the outer 50% of the enamel surface;

2 = demineralization (brown discolouration) involving between 50% of the enamel and one third of the dentine;

3 = demineralization (brown discolouration) involving the middle third of the dentine;

4 = demineralization (brown discolouration) involving the inner third of the dentine.

The histological scoring was carried out by two examiners concurrently. The two examiners re-scored 10 teeth and agreed the second time on 8 of the 10 scores. The percentages of tooth surfaces classified clinically with codes 0, 1, 2, 3, 4 and 5 + 6 and seen on sectioning to extend into dentine are presented in table 2. These data support the decision of the ICDAS II workshop to switch the original codes 3 and 4 (ICDAS I) to portray a sequential progression of dental caries.

The likelihood ratios (LR) that a tooth classified with codes 2, 3, 4 or 5 + 6 had dental caries into dentine, relative to a tooth classified with codes 0 or 1, are presented in table 3. These ratios show that the ICDAS II (with codes 3 and 4 switched) has an ordinal sequence in terms of histological extension into dentine. These ratios are relatively high compared with the LR of standard medical signs and symptoms. For example, in relation to heart attacks, an elevation in the ST segmentation on an electrocardiogram has an LR of 11.2, while radiating pain to both arms has an LR of 7.1 [53].

Ekstrand et al. [20] also investigated the relationship between the ICDAS I 7-point classification when applied to the occlusal, free smooth and approximal surfaces of

Table 2. Percentage of tooth surfaces classified using the ICDAS by histological caries status

Clinical code	Number of teeth	Percentage in dentine
0	2	0
1	11	9
2	18	50
3	8	88
4	13	77
5 + 6	5	100
Total	57	

Table 3. LR of ICDAS-I-classified teeth having caries in dentine

Histological	Clinical						Number
	0	1	2	3	4	5	
0	1	0	2	0	0	0	3
1	1	10	7	1	3	0	22
2			8	3	7	1	19
3		1		1	1	1	4
4			1	3	2	3	9
Total	2	11	18	8	13	5	57
LR (0–1)			6.5	11.4	10.0	13.0	

extracted posterior teeth. The results using the ICDAS I are cross-tabulated with the original histological scoring system [20]. A strong relationship was found between the two variables for occlusal, free smooth and approximal surfaces (Spearman correlation coefficients = 0.93, 0.95 and 0.94, respectively). Similarly for the second examiner, the correlation coefficients were 0.87, 0.96 and 0.92, respectively. The positive LR that an approximal lesion classified with ICDAS codes 3–6 is in dentine is around 18.

Recent work has included validation of the ICDAS criteria in the approximal surfaces of both permanent and primary teeth. Martignon et al. [54] conducted a study to determine the relationship between lesion severity assessed by ICDAS criteria and histological depth on sound and carious approximal surfaces of 140 permanent teeth and 108 primary teeth. A total of 160 carious or sound permanent proximal surfaces and 136 carious or sound primary proximal surfaces were finally assessed by the main investigator. The surfaces were cleaned and clinically assessed by means of a head light, WHO probes and air-drying. Re-examination of all teeth was conducted after 8 days. Afterwards teeth were cut longitudinally at the centre of the lesions and 220-μm-thick sections were stereomicroscopically assessed for demineralization by an independent examiner, as follows: 0 = no demineralization; 1 = enamel demineralization limited to the outer 50% of the enamel layer; 2 = demineralization involving 50% of the enamel to one third of the dentine; 3 = demineralization involving the middle third of the dentine, and 4 = demineralization involving the inner third of the dentine. Intra-examiner reproducibilities (κ) for the ICDAS scores were 0.86 and 0.92 for the permanent and the primary teeth, respectively. Spearman's correlation coefficient was 0.87 for the permanent teeth and 0.92 for the primary teeth. Results showed that the correlation between ICDAS scores and histological changes was excellent both for primary and permanent proximal lesions; intra-examiner reproducibility was also excellent.

Shoaib et al. [55] confirm these findings in the primary teeth in an in vitro study to assess the reproducibility of the detection of occlusal and approximal caries in primary teeth using the ICDAS II criteria. Three trained examiners independently examined 112 extracted primary molars under dental surgery conditions, using the ICDAS II criteria. The teeth were cleaned and set up in groups of 4, in pink impression putty to mimic their anatomical positions. The condition of the teeth used ranged from clinically sound to cavitated; extensively broken down teeth were excluded. As per the ICDAS II criteria, a 3:1 syringe and blunt probe were used during the examinations, and the most advanced lesion on each surface was scored. Each examination was conducted blind and repeated by each examiner after a gap of at least 24 h. κ values were calculated to assess reproducibility of the examinations. The intra-examiner reproducibility ranged from 0.74 to 0.83 and from 0.72 to 0.85, at the D_1 and ICDAS II codes 2/3 diagnostic thresholds, respectively. The inter-examiner reproducibility ranged from 0.60 to 0.72 and from 0.63 to 0.80 at the D1 and code 2/3 diagnostic thresholds. These values generally represent 'substantial agreement'. These researchers concluded that the reproducibility of the ICDAS II was acceptable when applied to primary molar teeth.

Inter- and intra-examiner reproducibility and accuracy in the detection and assessment of occlusal caries has been confirmed by Jablonski-Momeni et al. [56] in extracted teeth. In this study 4 dentists examined the occlusal surfaces of 100 teeth using the ICDAS II criteria, after which the teeth were serially sectioned and histologically assessed for the depth of caries. Three of the examiners were inexperienced in the use of ICDAS II prior to training by the 4th examiner. The weighted κ values for inter- and intra-examiner reproducibility were 0.62–0.83. Two classification systems for the histology were applied [20, 57], having a moderate to strong relationship to the ICDAS scores (r3 = 0.43–0.72). At the D_1 threshold of detection (enamel and dentinal caries), specificity was 0.74–0.91 and sensitivity 0.59–0.73 whilst at the D_3 threshold of detection (dentinal lesions only) specificity was 0.82–0.94 and sensitivity 0.48–0.83 for the 4 examiners.

Ismail et al. [58] have collected data on training of examiners in the Detroit Dental Health Project. The study found good to very good interexaminer reliability among US general dentists who were trained over a period of 1 week. The κ coefficients for interexaminer agreement ranged between 0.74 and 0.88. The intra-examiner κ coefficients for the two main examiners were around 0.78. One secondary examiner had an intra-examiner reliability of 0.77 and a 4th secondary examiner who worked only on Saturdays had an intra-examiner κ of 0.50. Details on reliability analysis using log-linear modelling are presented in a separate paper [58]. For caries adjacent to restorations and sealants, the interexaminer κ coefficient ranged between 0.33 for 1 examiner and over 0.80 for the 2 main examiners. The main examiners had an intra-examiner reliability of 0.80.

Ekstrand et al. [20] reported that intra-examiner κ coefficients when examining extracted teeth using the ICDAS I were substantial (κ = 0.87). The interexaminer reliability was around 0.80.

Data from the numerous studies at Indiana University have shown the ICDAS criteria to be a reliable and effective tool for various applications. It has been successfully applied in different types of studies, in vitro studies as well as clinical studies (validation study, secondary caries, epidemiology, study on caries risk factors and clinical trial), in different dentitions (primary and permanent teeth), in different age groups (children, teenagers, young adults, adults) and by multiple examiners with different backgrounds as well as previous exposure and experience with the criteria.

Several training and calibration studies have been conducted in Indiana and co-operative sites. The ICDAS criteria were used in a project in Mexico, where caries risk factors and indicators measured in 5 rural village populations were correlated with caries prevalence. Intra-examiner reliability gave a weighted κ of 0.93 [59].

International Caries Detection and Assessment System Comparability with Other Caries Detection Systems

The ICDAS codes were developed to allow backward comparability with other systems of caries detection such as the WHO basic methods [6]. Some interesting work has been done using these two criterion systems in parallel which demonstrated the additional caries yield found at the D_1 threshold of detection using the ICDAS [60]. Figure 12 gives a side-by-side comparison of ICDAS and WHO basic methods codes. It should be noted that the loose definition of the WHO Basic Methods codes has meant that there has been a difference in how the codes have been interpreted in different parts of the world, particularly in the threshold at which caries is recorded as present or absent. In particular there has been a great deal of variation between surveys and countries as to whether enamel cavitation (which would be ICDAS code 3)

Comparison between WHO[1] and ICDAS II[2] Codes		
WHO codes	**ICDAS II codes**	**Visual caries detection threshold**
0, A (sound)	00	Sound
	01	Non-cavitated — Enamel caries (visually)
	02	
	03	Surface discontinuity[3]
1, B (decayed crown)	04, 14, 24	Non-cavitated[4] — Obvious dentinal caries (visually)
	05, 15, 25, 80–85	Cavitated
	06, 16, 26, 86	
2, C (filled and decayed)	All 2-digit codes starting with 3, 4, 5, 6 and ending 4, 5, or 6	
3, D (filled, no decay)	All 2-digit codes starting with 3, 4, 5, 6 and ending 0, 1 or 3 (see exception below for crowns/abutments placed for reasons other than caries)	
4, E (missing due to caries)	97	
5 (permanent tooth missing for other reasons)	98	
6, F (sealant)	10, 20, 11, 21, 13, 23 – also WHO may include composite restorations restoring an investigated occlusal fissure to be in this category, i.e. some instances of codes 30, 31, 32, 33	
7, G (bridge abutment or special crown)	Any 2-digit code starting 6 and ending 0, 1, 2 or 3 and placed for some reason other than for caries, e.g. bridge abutment or because of trauma	
8 (unerupted)	99	

[1] Oral Surveys – Basic Methods, ed 4. http://www.whocollab.of.mah.se/expl/orhsurvey97.html (accessed December 14, 2007).

[2] ICDAS II codes http://www.icdas.org/ (accessed December 14, 2007).

[3] ICDAS II code 3 is enamel caries with surface discontinuity but no dentine is exposed. At the dentinal threshold for visual detection therefore this would be coded as sound even though it is known that many of these lesions would histologically involve dentine. Please note that interpretation of the WHO criteria varies internationally as to whether ICDAS code 3 lesions would be regarded as sound or not.

[4] There may be microcavitation but no cavity exposing dentine.

Fig. 12. Comparison between WHO codes and ICDAS.

should be coded as 'sound' or 'caries' leading to continuing difficulties in comparing between studies using WHO basic methods criteria.

Further Research and Priorities for Implementation

Priorities for Research

The ICDAS Foundation and the ICDAS Committee have been committed to defining a continuing research agenda, and this is a continuing task which is updated and revisited.

The clear priorities for research are the worldwide gaps in evidence around caries adjacent to restorations and sealants and around the reliable detection of caries in root surfaces.

Priorities for Implementation

There is a continuing international challenge to implement evidence that has been published and known for decades in this area. In some countries and systems, modern methods and approaches to clinical visual lesion detection to enable prevention-orientated caries management are well established. In other (often well-developed) countries and systems, the barriers to implementation are complex and remain strong. This area is itself a research priority as, at present in many countries, the dental profession can be accused of 'preferring to treat rather than prevent oral diseases' [61].

Implementation activities should be focussed on the different needs of the dental and public/stakeholder communities involved with caries, its prevention and management in the domains of clinical practice, research, public health and education. The continuing use of sharp explorers/probes without clinical benefit and the frequently limited knowledge about the dynamics of early carious lesions are priorities to overcome in many areas, but are generally accepted good practice in other locations.

References

1. Backer-Dirks O, van Amerongen J, Winkler KC: A reproducible method for caries evaluation. J Dent Res 1951;30:346–359.
2. Marthaler TM: A standardized system of recording dental conditions. Helv Odontol Acta 1966;10:1–19.
3. Soggnaes RF. The importance of a detailed clinical examination of carious lesions. J Dent Res 1940;19:11–15.
4. Radike AW: Criteria for diagnosis of dental caries; in: Proceedings of the Conference on the Clinical Testing of Cariostatic Agents, Oct 14–16, 1968. Chicago, American Dental Association, 1972, pp 87–88.
5. World Health Organization: Oral Health Surveys: Basic Methods, ed 2. Geneva, World Health Organization, 1977.
6. World Health Organization: Oral Health Surveys: Basic Methods, ed 4. Geneva, World Health Organization, 1997.
7. Pitts NB, Fyffe HE: The effect of varying diagnostic thresholds upon clinical caries data for a low prevalence group. J Dent Res 1988;67:592–596.
8. Ismail A, Vrodeur JM, Gagnon P, Payette M, Picard D, Hamalian T, et al: Prevalence of non-cavitated and cavitated carious lesions in a random sample of 7–9 year old schoolchildren in Montreal, Quebec. Community Dent Oral Epidemiol 1992;20:250–255.
9. Ekstrand KR, Ricketts DNJ, Kidd EAM, Qvist V, Schou S: Detection, diagnosing, monitoring and logical treatment of occlusal caries in relation to lesion activity and severity: an in vivo examination with histological validation. Caries Res 1998;32:247–254.
10. Fyffe HE, Deery CH, Nugent ZJ, Nuttall NM, Pitts NB: Effect of diagnostic threshold on the validity and reliability of epidemiological caries diagnosis using the Dundee Selectable Threshold Method for caries diagnosis (DSTM). Community Dent Oral Epidemiol.2000;28:42–51.
11. Nyvad B, Machiulskiene V, Baelum V: Reliability of a new caries diagnostic system differentiating between active and inactive caries lesions. Caries Res 1999;33:252–260.
12. Nyvad B, Machiulskiene V, Baelum V: Construct and predictive validity of clinical caries diagnostic criteria assessing lesion activity. J Dent Res 2003;82:117–122.
13. Nyvad B, ten Cate JM, Robinson C: Cariology in the 21st century – state of the art and future perspectives. Caries Res 2004;38:167–329.
14. Stookey G (ed): Proceedings of the First Annual Indiana Conference: Early Detection of Dental Caries. Indianapolis, Indiana University, 1996.
15. Stookey G (ed): Second International Conference on Detection of Early Caries. Indianapolis, Indiana University, 2000.
16. Stookey G (ed): Early Detection of Caries III. Indianapolis, Indiana University, 2004.

17 Pitts NB, Stamm J: International Consensus Workshop on Caries Clinical Trials (ICW-CCT) final consensus statements: agreeing where the evidence leads. J Dent Res 2004;83:125–128.

18 Ismail AI: Visual and visuo-tactile detection of dental caries. J Dent Res 2004;83(spec iss C):C56–C66.

19 Chesters RK, Pitts NB., Matuliene G, Kvedariene A, Huntington E, Bendinskaite R, Balciuniene I, Matheson J, Savage D. Milerience J: An abbreviated caries clinical trial design validated over 24 months. J Dent Res 2002;81:637–640.

20 Ekstrand KR, Ricketts DN, Kidd EA: Reproducibility and accuracy of three methods for assessment of demineralization depth of the occlusal surface: an in vitro examination. Caries Res 1997;31:224–231.

21 Ekstrand KR, Ricketts DN, Kidd EA. Occlusal caries: pathology, diagnosis and logical management. Dent Update 2001;28:380–387.

22 Ekstrand KR, Ricketts DNJ, Longbottom C, Pitts NB: Visual and tactile assessment of arrested initial enamel carious lesions: an in vivo pilot study. Caries Res 2005;39:173–177.

23 Ricketts DNJ, Ekstrand KR, Kidd EAM, Larsen T: Relating visual and radiographic ranked scoring systems for occlusal caries detection to histological and microbiological evidence. Operative Dent 2002;27:231–237.

24 Topping GVA, Hally JD, Bonner BC, Pitts NB: Training for the International Caries Detection and Assessment System (ICDAS II): CD-rom and web-based educational software. London, Smile-on, 2008.

25 Eggertsson H, Gudmundsdottir H, Agustsdottir H, Arnadottir IB, Eliasson ST, Saemundsson SR, Jonsson SH, Holbrook WP: Visual (ICDAS I) and radiographic detection of approximal caries in a national oral health survey (abstract 67). Caries Res 2007;41:292.

26 Bourgeois DM, Christensen LB, Ottolenghi L, Llodra JC, Pitts NB, Senakola E (eds): Health Surveillance in Europe – European Global Oral Health Indicators Development Project Oral Health Interviews and Clinical Surveys: Guidelines. Lyon, Lyon I University Press, 2008.

27 Ekstrand K, Qvist V, Thylstrup A: Light microscope study of the effect of probing in occlusal surfaces. Caries Res 1987;21:363–374.

28 Bergman G, Lindén LA: The action of the explorer on incipient caries. Svensk Tandläkare Tidsskrift 1969;62:629–634.

29 Ekstrand KR, Kuzmina I, Bjorndal L, Thylstrup A: Relationship between external and histologic features of progressive stages of caries in the occlusal fossa. Caries Res 1995;29:243–250.

30 Mjör IA, Toffenetti F: Secondary caries: a literature review with case reports. Quintessence Int 2000;31:165–179.

31 Tobi H, Kreulen CM, Vondeling H, van Amerongen WE: Cost-effectiveness of composite resins and amalgam in the replacement of amalgam class II restorations. Community Dent Oral Epidemiol 1999;27:137–143.

32 Miller WA, Massler M: Permeability and staining of active and arrested lesions in dentine. Br Dent J 1962;112:187–197.

33 Kidd EAM: Caries diagnosis within restored teeth. Oper Dent 1989;14:149–158.

34 Kidd EAM: Caries diagnosis within restored teeth; in Anusavice KJ (ed): Quality Evaluation of Dental Restorations: Criteria for Placement and Replacement. Chicago, Quintessence Publishing, 1989, pp 111–123.

35 Kidd EAM, Joyston BS, Beighton D: Diagnosis of secondary caries: a laboratory study. Br Dent J 1994;176:135–139.

36 Rudolphy MP, van Amerongen JP, Penning C, ten Cate JM: Grey discoloration and marginal fracture for the diagnosis of secondary caries in molars with occlusal amalgam restorations: an in vitro study. Caries Res 1995;29:371–376.

37 Topping GVA: Secondary Caries Misdiagnosis: An in vitro Study in Premolar and Molar Teeth Restored with Amalgam and Conjoint Analysis of Patients' and Dentists' Preferences for Attributes of a Caries Diagnosis Device; thesis, University of Dundee, 2001.

38 Kidd EAM, Joyston BS, Beighton D: Marginal ditching and staining as a predictor of secondary caries around amalgam restorations: a clinical and microbiological study. J Dent Res 1995;74:1206–1211.

39 Rudolphy MP, van Loveren C, van Amerongen JP: Grey discoloration for the diagnosis of secondary caries in teeth with class II amalgam restorations: an in vitro study. Caries Res 1996;30:189–193.

40 Bader JD, Shugars DA, Bonito AJ. Systematic review of selected dental caries diagnostic and management methods. J Dent Educ 2001;65:960–968.

41 Hix JO, O'Leary TJ: The relationship between cemental caries, oral hygiene status and fermentable carbohydrate intake. J Periodontol 1976;47:394–404.

42 Banting DW: Diagnosis and prediction of root caries. Adv Dent Res 1993;7:80–86.

43 Banting DW: The diagnosis of root caries. J Dent Educ 2001;65:991–996.

44 Katz RV: Development of an index for the prevalence of root caries. J Dent Res 1984;63:814–818.

45 US Department of Health and Human Services: Oral health of United States adults. NIH Publication No 87-2868. National Institutes of Health, 1987.
46 Warren JJ, Levy SM, Wefel JS: Explorer probing of root caries lesions. Spec Care Dent 2003;23:18–21.
47 Hellyer PH, Beighton D, Heath MR, Lynch EJR: Root caries in older people attending a general practice in East Sussex. Br Dent J 1990;169:201–206.
48 Lynch E, Beighton D: A comparison of primary root caries lesions classified according to color. Caries Res 1994;28:233–239.
49 Billings RJ, Brown LR, Kaster AG: Contemporary treatment strategies for root surface dental caries. Gerodontics 1985;1:20–27.
50 Beighton D, Lynch E, Heath MR: A microbiological study of primary root caries lesions with different treatment needs. J Dent Res 1993;63:623–629.
51 Hellyer P, Lynch E: The diagnosis of root caries. Gerodontology 1991;9:95–102.
52 Leake JL: Clinical decision-making for caries management in root caries. J Dent Educ 2001;65:1147–1153.
53 Panju AA, Hemmelgarn BR, Guyatt GH, Simel DL: The rational clinical examination: is this patient having a myocardial infarction? JAMA 1998;280:1256–1263.
54 Martignon S, Ekstrand K, Cuevas S, Reyes JF, Torres C, Tamayo M, Bautista G: Relationship between ICDAS II scores and histological lesion depth on proximal surfaces of primary and permanent teeth (abstract 61). Caries Res 2007;41:290.
55 Shoaib L, Deery C, Nugent ZN, Ricketts DNJ: Reproducibility of ICDAS II criteria for occlusal and approximal caries detection in primary teeth (abstract 63). Caries Res 2007;41:290.
56 Jablonski-Momeni A, Stachniss V, Ricketts DN, Heinzel-Gutenbrunner M: Reproducibility and accuracy of the ICDAS-II for detection of occlusal caries in vitro. Caries Res 2008;42:79–87.
57 Downer MC: Concurrent validity of an epidemiological diagnostic system for caries with histological appearance of extracted teeth as validating criterion. Caries Res 1975;9:231–246.
58 Ismail AI, Sohn W, Tellez M, Amaya A, Sen A, Hasson H, Pitts NB: Reliability of the International Caries Detection and Assessment System (ICDAS): an integrated system for measuring dental caries. Community Dent Oral Epidemiol 2007;35:170–178.
59 Cook SL, Martinez-Mier EA, Dean JA, Weddell JA, Sanders BJ, Eggertsson H, Ofner S, Yoder K: Dental caries experience and association to risk indicators of remote rural populations. Int J Paediatr Dentistry 2008;18:275–283.
60 Kuhnisch J, Berger S, Goddon I, Senkel H, Pitts N, Heinrich-Weltzien R: Occlusal caries detection in permanent molars according to WHO basic methods, ICDAS II and laser fluorescence measurements. Community Dent Oral Epidemiol 2008;36:475–484.
61 Editorial: Oral health: prevention is key. Lancet 2009;373:1.

G.V. A. Topping
Dental Health Services and Research Unit, University of Dundee
Mackenzie Building, Kirsty Semple Way
Dundee DD2 4BF (UK)
Tel. +44 1382 420067, Fax +44 1382 420051, E-Mail n.b.pitts@cpse.dundee.ac.uk

Traditional Lesion Detection Aids

K.W. Neuhaus[a] · R. Ellwood[b] · A. Lussi[a] · N.B. Pitts[c]

[a]Department of Preventive, Restorative and Pediatric Dentistry, School of Dental Medicine, University of Bern, Bern, Switzerland; [b]Dental Health Unit, Dental School, University of Manchester, Manchester, [c]Dental Health Services and Research Unit, University of Dundee, Dundee, UK

Abstract

Lesion detection aids ideally aim at increasing the sensitivity of visual caries detection without trading off too much in terms of specificity. The use of a dental probe (explorer), bitewing radiography and fibre-optic transillumination (FOTI) have long been recommended for this purpose. Today, probing of suspected lesions in the sense of checking the 'stickiness' is regarded as obsolete, since it achieves no gain of sensitivity and might cause irreversible tooth damage. Bitewing radiography helps to detect lesions that are otherwise hidden from visual examination, and it should therefore be applied to a new patient. The diagnostic performance of radiography at approximal and occlusal sites is different, as this relates to the 3-dimensional anatomy of the tooth at these sites. However, treatment decisions have to take more into account than just lesion extension. Bitewing radiography provides additional information for the decision-making process that mainly relies on the visual and clinical findings. FOTI is a quick and inexpensive method which can enhance visual examination of all tooth surfaces. Both radiography and FOTI can improve the sensitivity of caries detection, but require sufficient training and experience to interpret information correctly. Radiography also carries the burden of the risks and legislation associated with using ionizing radiation in a health setting and should be repeated at intervals guided by the individual patient's caries risk. Lesion detection aids can assist in the longitudinal monitoring of the behaviour of initial lesions.

Copyright © 2009 S. Karger AG, Basel

Probing

The act of clinical caries detection was traditionally supported by a dental mirror, optimal light and a sharp-ended explorer (in some countries referred to as a probe). The resistance to withdrawal or 'stickiness' of a probe forced gently, moderately or even firmly into a suspected fissure or pit was expected to be correlated with the presence of tooth decay [for a review, see 1]. More recently in many parts of the world the use of a sharp probe has been discouraged for two main reasons. Firstly, it does not seem to provide any benefit over and above that provided by meticulous visual examination of a dry tooth and does not increase sensitivity or specificity [2]. For non-cavitated

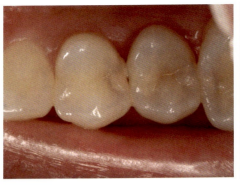 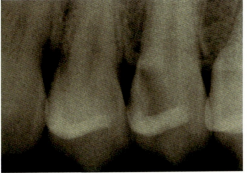

Fig. 1. Diagnosis in adjacent teeth. **a** Approximal lesion at the distal aspect. **b** Corresponding radiograph.

lesions, the reported sensitivity of visual inspection combined with probing is as low as 14% [3] to 24% [4]. Secondly, probing has been shown to irreversibly damage the tooth, turning a sound, remineralizable subsurface lesion into a cavitated lesion much more prone to lesion progression [5–7]. In addition there has been theoretical concern regarding bacterial cross-infection via probing from one site to another [8]. For epidemiological surveys, the WHO recommends the use of a round-ended periodontal probe for caries detection [9]. The use of a sharp probe to detect surface roughness by gently stroking across the tooth surface may have some relevance for the assessment of lesion activity (R_w; see Ekstrand et al. [this vol., pp. 63–90]) [10]. Not using a sharp explorer for coronal lesion detection by sticking it into pits and fissures, but instead performing meticulous visual inspection [see the chapter by Topping and Pitts, this vol., pp. 15–41]) in combination with other non-invasive caries detection aids is highly recommended (R_s). However, for root caries assessment or during excavation, a probe can render good and necessary information on tissue softness.

Radiography

In a clinical setting, a true tooth-by-tooth diagnosis might be hampered in adjacent teeth, when one lesion is obviously present. In figure 1a, one can clearly distinguish an approximal lesion at the distal aspect of tooth 24, which looks larger than tooth 25. On the corresponding radiograph (fig. 1b), one might be surprised to see a much larger dentinal caries at the mesial aspect of tooth 25. Only on careful examination might one see a significant gradual change of colour in tooth 25. Radiography helps to overcome this phenomenon of restricted visual perception in a quick and easy way. Therefore, apart from probing, radiography is the most widespread lesion detection aid, particularly with respect to otherwise invisible or poorly visible approximal areas.

Table 1. Possible factors influencing the diagnostic quality of bitewing radiography

Processing step	Possible confounders	Possible refinements
Film	storage	upright and cool storage
	film type	
	film processing	fresh developing chemicals
		correct temperature
		cautious handling of the film
	film contrast	
X-ray	radiation dose	regular consistency tests
	exposure time	
	angulation	beam-aiming device
Tooth	correct positioning of the film	film holder
	white-spot lesions may appear to be deep enamel lesions	anatomical knowledge
	Mach band effect	
	'burn-out'	
	triangular-shaped radiolucency	
Examiner	individual experience	
	viewing conditions	magnification, viewing kit

Radiography always carries risks associated with the use of ionizing radiation, some risks are amenable to reduction, others are a statistical event beyond control. For these reasons there is an onus on all health professionals to reduce or eliminate radiation exposures. In order to reduce the radiation dose over periapical and tomographic views, and because of superior imaging geometry for visualizing caries, for detection purposes the bitewing technique is the most commonly used method. The clinical crowns and the alveolar ridge on one side are projected on a film or digital sensor (size 3 × 4 cm). In children, due to a shorter clinical crown, the projection also often allows diagnosis of the periradicular region (film size 2 × 3 cm). From a risk:benefit perspective, it is clearly important to extract as much other information as possible from a bitewing radiograph, that is to include both the periodontium and the endodontium where possible.

A correct radiographic diagnosis depends on the correct performance of crucial steps and contains a variety of factors which influence the diagnostic outcome (table 1).

Diagnostic Performance of Dental Radiography
The sensitivities for the radiographic detection of both approximal and occlusal dentinal lesions are quite high, compared to clinical visual detection, in in vitro settings

(50–70%) [for reviews, see 11, 12]. Generally, it is possible to detect approximal lesions earlier than with visual diagnosis alone [13]. However, the validity of detecting enamel caries is limited on the approximal surfaces and low for the occlusal aspect. This difference relates to the 3-dimensional anatomy of the tooth at these sites where on the 2-dimensional radiograph, the superimposed cuspal tissues obscure early changes in the occlusal fissures. There are some differing views linked to study methodology in that many studies show that radiographic detection is of value on occlusal surfaces [14, 15], while a study in a population of Lithuanian children with high caries rates revealed that bitewing radiography was only of limited value compared to visual inspection on the occlusal aspect but yielded better results for approximal dentinal lesions [16]. Another important aspect is the caries prevalence of the individuals under study. In an in vivo study comparing visual-tactile detection with bitewing radiography in a low-caries-prevalence cohort of 168 adolescents aged 14 years, bitewing radiography was more sensitive than visual-tactile inspection for both the occlusal and the approximal aspects [17]. However, the diagnostic error of false-positive results was purported to be high in this population, and the value of bitewing screening was questioned. If the caries prevalence is low (i.e. the number of sound surfaces is high), a more sensitive method with slightly smaller specificity is bound to produce larger numbers of false-positive data, which, as a consequence, may result in too early invasive treatment [18].

Bitewing – Digital or Conventional?

The accuracy of conventional and digital bitewing radiography is comparable and shows no statistically significant difference [19]; this is despite often expressed user preference for conventional film images which is probably related to familiarity with the traditional image. There are numerous arguments in favour of digital bitewings: they are less time consuming, potentially require lower doses of ionizing radiation (but sensor size and number of exposures have to be taken into account to reach valid comparisons) and offer options of digitally enhancing contrast or optical density changes. This capability was shown to increase the number of correctly detected occlusal non-cavitated dentinal lesions compared to visual inspection, conventional radiography and xeroradiographs [20]. However, depending on the digital system used, a connecting wire with the intra-oral sensor might interfere with the correct positioning of the film, or the effective radiation field may be smaller [21]. Furthermore, the 'printouts' of digital radiography render pictures of lower quality. The use of digital radiography in a private clinical setting is however probably more influenced by individual economic aspects than by its clinical performance. With the recent technological advances in sensor design as has happened in photography, it is likely that the performance of these systems will soon be significantly improved further, and this, combined with the opportunities to digitally enhance radiographs by image processing, will almost certainly make this the imaging medium of choice in the near future.

Frequencies of Taking Bitewing Radiographs

The frequency of taking radiographic images depends on the individual caries risk [15], lesion activity and on the individual benefit to a patient: the lower the individual's caries risk, the lower the frequency of bitewing radiography required. But, if the caries risk is high, all tooth surfaces can be examined by visual inspection or other non-ionizing caries detection tools with satisfactory diagnostic performance; taking frequent radiographs is obviously not necessary. The present evidence on the balance of risk and benefit indicates that the diagnostic yield for caries diagnosis is high enough to justify individualized examinations, particularly as changes in the morphology of caries have rendered clinical diagnosis of dentinal lesions less sensitive (although this issue must be kept under review as alternative diagnostic technologies develop). There is good evidence that initial posterior bitewing radiographs are required for all new dentate patients over 5 years of age with posterior teeth. This procedure is required as an adjunct to clinical examination for the detection of caries on both the approximal and occlusal surfaces of the teeth. Although a 'blanket' regimen of routine radiographic examination at fixed intervals cannot be advocated, individualized bitewing examinations at varying frequencies determined on the basis of caries risk are supported [15]. The guidelines of the European Academy of Paediatric Dentistry [22] recommend radiography intervals of 1 year for patients with a high caries risk and 2–4 years for low-risk patients (R_e). However, earlier recommendations [23] as well as the European guidelines on radiation protection in dental radiology [24] aim at half-year intervals of bitewing radiography in high-risk patients. Another recommendation took into account the varying caries risk at different ages as well as the likelihood of lesion progression of children and teenagers in areas with low caries prevalence [25]. The ages of 5, 8–9, 12–14 and 15–16 years were identified as key ages at which to take bitewing radiographs. However, it remains a major task in dentistry to identify the subjects prone to faster lesion progression in order to apply the most appropriate timing of radiography. New patients (aged 5 years or more) unknown to the dentist should receive bitewing radiographs in order to obtain baseline information (R_e).

Interpretation of Radiographic Data

Bitewing radiography tends to be associated with a relatively high proportion of false-positive scores (3–30%) [12]. This is due to the fact that radiography projects a 3-dimensional object on a 2dimensional layer, thus superimposing differently mineralized and radiolucent tissues. For this reason it is important that radiographs are interpreted in the clinical setting. False-positive data might result from the Mach band effect (which is an inclination to see a radiolucency in the dentine-enamel junction where no dentinal lesion is actually present [26]), from the burn-out effect (radiolucencies at the cemento-enamel junction) or triangular-shaped radiolucencies (due to prominent palatal cusps together with reduced mesial crown diameters [27]). These effects are perceptual phenomena enhancing the contrast between a dark and a relatively lighter area which is sharply demarcated [28]. Besides, another complicating factor could be explained by the fact that caries lesions located in pits and fissures might be superimposed onto the dentine radiographically due to the complex anatomy of the occlusal area [26]. Dental radiography also shows the tendency to underestimate lesion extension into dentine (fig. 2).

Due to the complexity of individual caries risk assessment [see the chapter by Twetman and Fontana, this vol., pp. 91–101] and dental radiographic procedures themselves requiring subjective interpretation of the radiographic images, the degree of correct processing of information will be substantially influenced by the observer's training and experience [29]. A higher sensitivity paired with lower specificity and lower interexaminer agreement can be expected from untrained dentists [30].

Treatment Decisions Based on Radiography
The detection of the presence of an approximal cavity is subject to visual inspection, sometimes only after temporary tooth separation [18]. In scanning electron microscopy enlargement, 97% of approximal surfaces of lesions radiographically extending only into the outer enamel were shown to have microcavities and surface discontinuities [31]. However, in a clinical setting Pitts and Rimmer [32] found that for approximal lesions radiographically extending into the outer dentine 59% of the surfaces of permanent molars and more than 70% of the surfaces of deciduous molars were still intact. On radiographs, the presence of a cavity can only be estimated from lesion extension into dentine, resulting in more 'aggressive' (over)treatment the nearer the cut-off for invasive intervention is placed to the tooth surface [33–35]. Since lesion progression is dependent on the continuing presence of viable bacteria, and lesion arrestment is dependent on the capability of constantly removing them, a treatment decision must not only rely on radiographic lesion extension, but also has to take clinical factors into account (R_s). Lesion behaviour over time can be monitored by serial bitewing radiographs, which can be used to assess success or otherwise preventive treatment options applied to initial lesions [15].

Digital caries detection software was designed to support the treatment decision based on bitewing radiography. While the inventor found a good correlation between cavitated lesions and analysis results [36], these findings could not be supported in an independent trial [37]. Therefore, today, despite computer-aided image analysis of radiolucencies having been shown to be a viable proposition more than 20 years ago [38], it is still too early to rely on statistical caries detection software computing cavitation probabilities, but future developments are to be awaited.

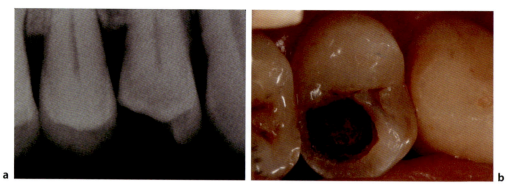

Fig. 2. Lesion extension into dentine. **a** Radiograph. **b** Clinical assessment.

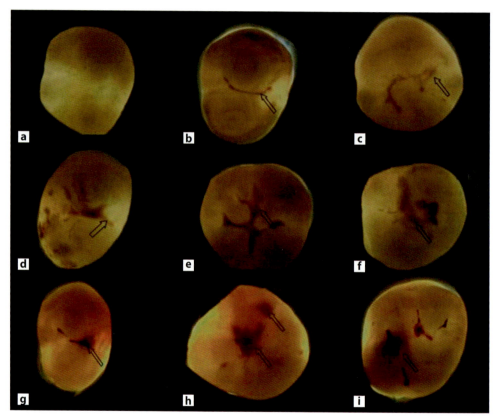

Fig. 3. **a** Sound tooth, note clean fissure morphology. **b** Stained fissure, no widening of fissure pattern when transilluminated (arrow). **c** Slight widening of fissure pattern (arrow) when transilluminated indicating demineralization. Similar in appearance to ICDAS code 1 lesion. **d** Widening of fissure pattern (arrow) indicating hypomineralization. Similar in appearance to ICDAS code 2 lesion. **e** As above. **f** Microcavitated lesion with orange discolouration at the base of the fissure (arrow) indicating penetration into dentine. Similar in appearance to ICDAS code 3 lesion. **g** Dentine shadow (arrow) with FOTI demonstrating orange and grey discolouration. Similar in appearance to ICDAS code 3–4 lesion. **h** As above. **i** Dentine shadow (arrow) with FOTI, demonstrating orange and grey discolouration. Similar in appearance to ICDAS code 4 lesion.

Fibre-Optic Transillumination

The method of tooth transillumination with an appropriate intense light source is widely accepted by dental practitioners for caries detection in anterior teeth. For this purpose, transillumination is easy, fast and inexpensive.

Fibre-optic transillumination (FOTI) uses the principle of light scattering to increase contrast between normal and carious enamel. Light is applied to the side of the tooth and its transmission observed from either the opposing side, or occlusally in the case of molars and premolars. As light is scattered more in demineralized enamel than sound enamel, a lesion appears dark on a light background. In addition to this, carious dentine appears orange, brown or grey underneath the enamel, and this can significantly aid discrimination between enamel and dentinal lesions. FOTI provides a 3-dimensional view of the tooth and the caries within. This can provide a significant benefit in restorative dentistry enabling cavity preparation to remain minimally invasive. FOTI has not been adopted widely in dental practice, probably because of difficulties in obtaining suitable equipment. To facilitate light transmission through the tooth, high-intensity illuminators are required and to detect smaller lesions, particularly approximally, point sources of illumination are desirable. More recently high-intensity LED light sources have provided a cheap and more widely available source of equipment.

Most of the early FOTI research concentrated on the detection of proximal lesions, and the performance with respect to this has been reviewed by Vaarkamp et al. [39]. It was concluded that the specificity of both FOTI and bitewing radiography was high but that the sensitivity of FOTI was significantly lower than bitewing radiography. In another study [40], detection of approximal dentinal lesions using clinical examination, FOTI and bitewing radiographs were compared in vitro. All specificity values exceeded 0.95 with sensitivities for clinical examination of 0.38, bitewing of 0.59 and FOTI of 0.67 with no statistically significant difference between FOTI and bitewing radiography. It was concluded in this study, which demonstrates the upper range of reported performance, that the validity of FOTI can be at least as high as that of bitewing radiography, and that both were superior to unaided clinical diagnosis. However, proper training is needed in order to obtain such high levels of sensitivity and specificity [40], and some examiners find it extremely difficult to visualize and classify the shadows within teeth consistently. Several other studies render varying results for sensitivity ranging from 50 to 85% [39, 41]. Sensitivity for dentinal lesions is higher than for enamel lesions [42]. In the limited data available for digital FOTI, where the human eye is replaced by a CCD sensor, the ability of this method to detect incipient caries was limited [43]. In addition to use with approximal lesions, FOTI has also been more recently used for the detection of enamel and dentinal occlusal caries in combination with an enhanced visual examination (fig. 3) [44]. For enamel lesions, the diagnostic performance was similar for visual and FOTI examinations. However, the performance in the detection of dentine lesions was significantly improved with the adoption of the FOTI method. Differences between studies as with many methods may be the result of using inadequate equipment or insufficient training. As FOTI is non-invasive and does not use ionizing radiation, its use should be encouraged (R_e). FOTI is likely to support ad hoc decision-making in dental practice but is not as capable of monitoring caries lesions in the same way as bitewing radiography [15]. Moreover, concerning incomplete tooth fractures, FOTI is an invaluable tool for detecting enamel cracks [45].

References

1 Ismail AI: Visual and visuo-tactile detection of dental caries. J Dent Res 2004;83(spec iss C):56–66.
2 Lussi A: Validity of diagnostic and treatment decisions of fissure caries. Caries Res 1991;25:296–303.
3 Lussi A: Comparison of different methods for the diagnosis of fissure caries without cavitation. Caries Res 1993;27:409–416.
4 Penning C, van Amerongen JP, Seef RE, ten Cate JM: Validity of probing for fissure caries diagnosis. Caries Res 1992;26:445–449.
5 Ekstrand K, Qvist V, Thylstrup A: Light microscope study of the effect of probing in occlusal surfaces. Caries Res 1987;21:368–374.
6 Kühnisch J, Dietz W, Stösser L, Hickel R, Heinrich-Weltzien R: Effects of dental probing on occlusal surfaces – a scanning electron microscopy evaluation. Caries Res 2007;41:43–48.
7 Yassin OM: In vitro studies of the effect of a dental explorer on the formation of an artificial carious lesion. ASDC J Dent Child 1995;62:111–117.
8 Loesche WJ, Svanberg ML, Pape HR: Intraoral transmission of *Streptococcus mutans* by a dental explorer. J Dent Res 1979;58:1765–1770.
9 World Health Organization: Oral Health Surveys: Basic Methods. Geneva, WHO, 1997, pp 41–42.
10 Nyvad B, Machiulskiene V, Baelum V: Reliability of a new caries diagnostic system differentiating between active and inactive caries lesions. Caries Res 1999; 33:252–260.
11 Wenzel A: Bitewing and digital bitewing radiography for detection of caries lesions. J Dent Res 2004;83(spec iss C):72–75.
12 Wenzel A: Current trends in radiographic caries imaging. Oral Surg Oral Med Oral Pathol Oral Radiol Endod 1995;80:527–539.
13 Bloemendal E, de Vet HC, Bouter LM: The value of bitewing radiographs in epidemiological caries research: a systematic review of the literature. J Dent 2004;32:255–264.
14 Kidd EAM, Ricketts DNJ, Pitts NB: Occlusal caries diagnosis: a changing challenge for clinicians and epidemiologists. J Dent 1993;21:323–331.
15 Pitts NB: The use of bitewing radiographs in the management of dental caries: scientific and practical considerations. Dentomaxillofac Radiol 1996;25: 5–16.
16 Machiulskiene V, Nyvad B, Baelum V: A comparison of clinical and radiographic caries diagnoses in posterior teeth of 12-year-old Lithuanian children. Caries Res 1999;33:340–348.
17 Hintze H, Wenzel A: Clinically undetected dental caries assessed by bitewing screening in children with little caries experience. Dentomaxillofac Radiol 1994;23:19–23.
18 Hintze H, Wenzel A, Danielsen B, Nyvad B: Reliability of visual examination, fibre-optic transillumination, and bite-wing radiography, and reproducibility of direct visual examination following tooth separation for the identification of cavitated carious lesions in contacting approximal surfaces. Caries Res 1998;32:204–209.
19 Haak R, Wicht MJ, Noack MJ: Conventional, digital and contrast-enhanced bitewing radiographs in the decision to restore approximal carious lesions. Caries Res 2001;35:193–199.
20 Wenzel A, Larsen MJ, Fejerskov O: Detection of occlusal caries without cavitation by visual inspection, film radiographs, xeroradiographs, and digitized radiographs. Caries Res 1991;25:365–371.
21 Bahrami G, Hagström C, Wenzel A: Bitewing examination with four digital receptors. Dentomaxillofac Radiol 2003;32:317–321.
22 Espelid I, Mejàre I, Weerheijm K: EAPD guidelines for use of radiographs in children. Eur J Paediatr Dent 2003;4:40–48.
23 Pitts NB, Kidd EA: The prescription and timing of bitewing radiography in the diagnosis and management of dental caries: contemporary recommendations. Br Dent J 1992;172:225–257.
24 European Communities: European guidelines for radiation protection in dental radiology (issue 136). 2004. http://www.europa.eu.int (accessed December 23, 2008).

25 Mejàre I: Bitewing examination to detect caries in children and adolescents – when and how often? Dent Update 2005;32:588–590, 593–594, 596–597.
26 Espelid I, Tveit AB, Fjelltveit A: Variations among dentists in radiographic detection of occlusal caries. Caries Res 1994;28:169–175.
27 Kühnisch J, Pasler FA, Bucher K, Hickel R, Heinrich-Weltzien R: Frequency of non-carious triangular-shaped radiolucencies on bitewing radiographs. Dentomaxillofac Radiol 2008;37:23–27.
28 Berry HM Jr: Cervical burnout and Mach band: two shadows of doubt in radiologic interpretation of carious lesions. J Am Dent Assoc 1983;106:622–625.
29 Mileman PA, van den Hout WB: Comparing the accuracy of Dutch dentists and dental students in the radiographic diagnosis of dentinal caries. Dentomaxillofac Radiol 2002;31:7–14.
30 Lazarchik DA, Firestone AR, Heaven TJ, Filler SJ, Lussi A: Radiographic evaluation of occlusal caries: effect of training and experience. Caries Res 1995;29:355–358.
31 Kielbassa AM, Paris S, Lussi A, Meyer-Lueckel H: Evaluation of cavitations in proximal caries lesions at various magnification levels in vitro. J Dent 2006;34:817–822.
32 Pitts NB, Rimmer PA: An in vivo comparison of radiographic and directly assessed clinical caries status of posterior approximal surfaces in primary and permanent teeth. Caries Res 1992;26:146–152.
33 Domejean-Orliaguet S, Tubert-Jeannin S, Riordan PJ, Espelid I, Tveit AB: French dentists' restorative treatment decisions. Oral Health Prev Dent 2004;2:125–131.
34 Tveit AB, Espelid I, Skodje F: Restorative treatment decisions on approximal caries in Norway. Int Dent J 1999;49:165–172.
35 Mejàre I, Gröndahl HG, Carlstedt K, Grevér AC, Ottosson E: Accuracy at radiography and probing for the diagnosis of proximal caries. Scand J Dent Res 1985;93:178–184.
36 Gakenheimer DC: The efficacy of a computerized caries detector in intraoral digital radiography. J Am Dent Assoc 2002;133:883–890.
37 Wenzel A, Hintze H, Kold LM, Kold S: Accuracy of computer-automated caries detection in digital radiographs compared with human observers. Eur J Oral Sci 2002;110:199–203.
38 Pitts NB, Renson CE: Image analysis of bitewing radiographs: a histologically validated comparison with visual assessments of radiolucency depth in enamel. Br Dent J 1986;160:205–209.
39 Vaarkamp J, ten Bosch JJ, Verdonschot EH, Bronkhoorst EM: The real performance of bitewing radiography and fiber-optic transillumination in approximal caries diagnosis. J Dent Res 2000;79:1747–1751.
40 Peers A, Hill FJ, Mitropoulos CM, Holloway PJ: Validity and reproducibility of clinical examination, fibre-optic transillumination, and bite-wing radiology for the diagnosis of small approximal carious lesions: an in vitro study. Caries Res 1993;27:307–311.
41 Verdonschot EH, Bronkhorst EM, Wenzel A: Approximal caries diagnosis using fiber-optic transillumination: a mathematical adjustment to improve validity. Community Dent Oral Epidemiol 1991;19:329–332.
42 Holt RD, Azevedo MR: Fibre-optic transillumination and radiographs in diagnosis of approximal caries in primary teeth. Community Dent Health 1989;6:239–247.
43 Ando M. Performance of digital imaging fiber-optic transillumination (DIFOTI) for detection of non-cavitated primary caries. 7th Annu Indiana Conf, Indianapolis, 2006.
44 Cortes DF, Ellwood RP, Ekstrand KR: An in vitro comparison of a combined FOTI/visual examination of occlusal caries with other caries diagnostic methods and the effect of stain on their diagnostic performance. Caries Res 2003;37:8–16.
45 Ellis SG: Incomplete tooth fracture – proposal for a new definition. Br Dent J 2001;190:424–428.

Dr. Klaus W. Neuhaus
Department of Preventive, Restorative and Pediatric Dentistry, School of Dental Medicine
University of Bern, Freiburgstrasse 7
CH–3010 Bern (Switzerland)
Tel. +41 31 632 4974, Fax +41 31 632 9875, E-Mail klaus-neuhaus@zmk.unibe.ch

Novel Lesion Detection Aids

K.W. Neuhaus[a] · C. Longbottom[b] · R. Ellwood[c] · A. Lussi[a]

[a]Department of Preventive, Restorative and Pediatric Dentistry, School of Dental Medicine, University of Bern, Bern, Switzerland; [b]Dental Health Services and Research Unit, University of Dundee, Dundee, [c]Dental Health Unit, Dental School, University of Manchester, Manchester, UK

Abstract

Several non-invasive and novel aids for the detection of (and in some cases monitoring of) caries lesions have been introduced in the field of 'caries diagnostics' over the last 15 years. This chapter focusses on those available to dentists at the time of writing; continuing research is bound to lead to further developments in the coming years. Laser fluorescence is based on measurements of back-scattered fluorescence of a 655-nm light source. It enhances occlusal and (potentially) approximal lesion detection and enables semi-quantitative caries monitoring. Systematic reviews have identified false-positive results as a limitation. Quantitative light-induced fluorescence is another sensitive method to quantitatively detect and measure mineral loss both in enamel and some dentine lesions; again, the trade-offs with lower specificity when compared with clinical visual detection must be considered. Subtraction radiography is based on the principle of digitally superimposing two radiographs with exactly the same projection geometry. This method is applicable for approximal surfaces and occlusal caries involving dentine but is not yet widely available. Electrical caries measurements gather either site-specific or surface-specific information of teeth and tooth structure. Fixed-frequency devices perform best for occlusal dentine caries but the method has also shown promise for lesions in enamel and other tooth surfaces with multi-frequency approaches. All methods require further research and further validation in well-designed clinical trials. In the future, they could have useful applications in clinical practice as part of a personalized, comprehensive caries management system.

Copyright © 2009 S. Karger AG, Basel

Laser Fluorescence

Laser fluorescence (LF) has increasingly been adopted in the caries detection procedure for the last decade. In the Diagnodent device (Kavo, Biberach, Germany), a 655-nm monochromatic light is emitted from an optical tip/sensor, which can also detect the amount of back-scattered fluorescence [1]. During the caries detection procedure, the light beam enters the enamel and will either go unhindered to the dentine or be partially scattered. A regular crystalline structure like mature enamel is more

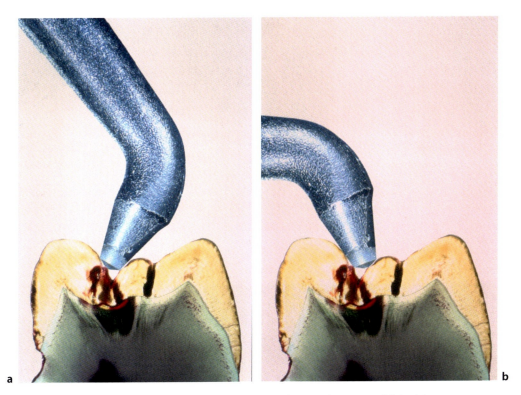

Fig. 1. a In LF measurements, the correct angulation of the probe is crucial. **b** In this case, a wrong angulation of the probe leads to false-negative readings.

transparent; thus, light can pass through the enamel layer with only little deflection. If the enamel layer is more inhomogeneous, more light will be diffracted and scattered. The scattered portion of the light then excites either the dental hard substance itself (and renders a measurement of the tooth's autofluorescence) or excites so-called fluorophores within the lesion. Fluorophores are particles with the property of fluorescing when excited by a specific wavelength of electromagnetic energy. In the case of 655 nm, the fluorescing particles have been identified as bacterial protoporphyrins [2, 3]. Thus, when a critically increased pore volume is exceeded, the amount of back-scattered fluorescence is – theoretically – proportional to the amount of bacterial infection, pore volume and lesion depth.

The measurements on the Diagnodent display render values between 0 (minimum fluorescence) and 99 (maximum fluorescence), thus theoretically making quantitative caries monitoring possible (fig. 1a, b). The manufacturer's instructions make clear, however, that only certain limited ranges can be used for assessing lesion extent, that there is overlap between some of these bands and that values over 45 may not be diagnostically useful. A more recently developed LF device (Diagnodent pen) provides 2 tips for both occlusal and approximal caries assessment (fig. 2, 3), although data supporting approximal detection on contacting teeth in vitro and in vivo is very limited at present.

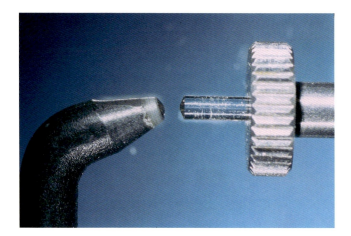

Fig. 2. The old Diagnodent and the occlusal tip of the Diagnodent pen have the same size and diameter.

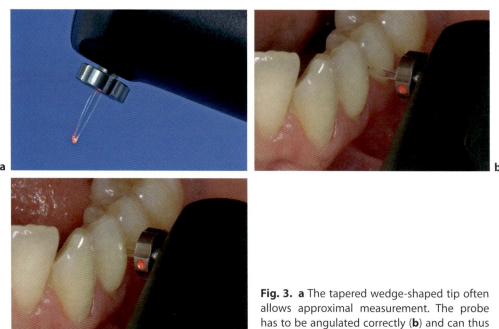

Fig. 3. a The tapered wedge-shaped tip often allows approximal measurement. The probe has to be angulated correctly (**b**) and can thus be introduced into the proximal space (**c**).

To date, many in vitro studies as well as an increasing number of in vivo clinical trials have been undertaken to validate the aforementioned general principle of detecting caries with LF. Generally, in vitro studies using teeth that were not frozen may be considered to be biased, because of a significant drop of the fluorescence signals due to degradation of porphyrins [4]. Narrative and systematic reviews have shown that LF is more sensitive on the occlusal aspect of posterior teeth than traditional diagnostic methods, but that specificity is inferior to clinical visual examination [5–7]. Both in vitro and in vivo studies show that the LF devices have a good intra- and interexaminer reproducibility [8–11]. In a randomized, clinical 2-centre study, the discrimination capability of LF between teeth with no apparent caries and carious teeth and between teeth with no obvious dentine caries and with dentine caries ranged from very good to moderate [11].

Extending the clinical use of LF has been explored in many studies: detecting recurrent caries [12, 13], residual caries during excavation [14], caries around orthodontic appliances [15, 16], root caries [17], caries under sealants [18, 19] as well as detection of subgingival calculus [20] have been described although in some studies the diagnostic utility is not clear against any reference standard. The initial simulated (in vitro) results of the newly proposed tip for the detection of approximal caries are promising, yet need to be verified in in vivo studies as well [9] (R_w). The width of this approximal tip (0.4 mm) might still be too large to assess all clinical interproximal areas. Yet, smaller diameters might result in a higher probability of mechanical instability and breakage and may therefore not be clinically applicable.

However, with both devices it must be appreciated that the value of the autofluorescence of the tooth itself has to be measured at the correct aspect of the tooth before readings of suspect tooth sites are taken [21]; this measurement has to be subtracted by the device from the measurement assessed at the lesion. Failure to carry out this procedure properly will compromise the validity and reproducibility of the results.

It is also essential to consider certain confounding factors, which might further contribute to false-positive readings in clinical practice. These include: the presence of stain [22], polishing pastes [23] or adjacent filling materials [24]. That is why prior to LF measurements, the tooth has to be cleaned professionally and dried. The clinical evidence for occlusal caries detection with LF is stronger than that for approximal caries detection; similarly, the detection performance for deep enamel or dentine caries is stronger than for shallow initial lesions. Due to the varied nature and quality of the studies reported in the literature, as well as the heterogeneity of the results and the range of comparators used, it is not possible to make a specific recommendation linked to the strength of evidence. The property of LF to rapidly and semi-quantitatively assess lesions has contributed to its widespread use in private dental practices and illustrates that dentists are looking for novel aids to help improve lesion detection. However, based on the research evaluations to date, LF should not be regarded as a stand-alone diagnostic tool but should instead be used as a second opinion in the decision-making process of caries diagnosis.

Quantitative Light-Induced Fluorescence

Quantitative light-induced fluorescence (QLF) is based on the principle that excitation of dentine with blue light (370 nm) causes it to fluoresce in the yellow-green region. By using a yellow high-pass filter (λ ≥540 nm) to cut out the excitation light, this fluorescence can be observed. When a lesion is present on the surface, an increase in light scattering is observed relative to the surrounding enamel. This has two important effects: firstly less excitation light reaches the dentine so that less fluorescence is produced underneath the lesion and secondly fluorescence that occurs is scattered through the lesion so that less light is observed. The net result of this is that the contrast between sound enamel and a lesion is improved with the lesion seen as being dark on a light green background. In addition to green fluorescence from dentine, bacterial porphyrins will fluoresce red.

This fluorescence method was developed for intra-oral quantification of mineral loss in enamel lesions using a *quantitative laser fluorescence* with a laser source and a colour microvideo CCD camera and computed image analysis (Inspektor Research Systems, the Netherlands) [25]. Some years earlier, the potential to use a light (rather than laser) source for endoscopically viewed filtered fluorescence for the clinical detection of carious lesions in enamel had been shown, the use of a video camera to acquire the images demonstrated and comparison made between endoscopic and conventional methods of caries diagnosis [26, 27]. The subtraction of digital fluorescence images of the caries lesion from fluorescence images of the surrounding enamel in QLF software enables the calculation of 3 lesion quantities: fluorescence loss (mean ΔF or ΔF_{max}), the area of the lesion (in square millimetres) and their product.

To facilitate clinical application, a small, portable system for intra-oral use was developed [28]. Data are collected, stored and analysed by custom-made software. The portable QLF device was validated against microradiographic and chemical analyses for the assessment of mineral changes in enamel and compared with results from measurements with the laser light equipment [28]. It was concluded that QLF was a sensitive, reproducible method for quantification of incipient enamel lesions limited to a depth of about 400 μm. Nevertheless, initial attempts to establish suitable cut-offs for dentine lesions were also made [29].

The in vivo reliability of QLF appears excellent for the quantification of smooth-surface initial caries, with intraclass correlation coefficients for interexaminer reproducibility of r = 0.95–0.99 [30, 31]. The QLF method has been applied in a few clinical studies. In some recent studies, QLF was used to test the natural behaviour of white-spot lesions after removal of orthodontic appliances [32, 33]. Six months after debonding, lesions with ΔF >10% improved to a greater extent than lesions with ΔF <10% [32], but 2 years after debonding those lesions did not improve significantly [33]. It was concluded in this study that QLF is appropriate for in vivo monitoring of mineral changes in white-spot enamel lesions and may be useful for the evaluation of preventive measures in caries-susceptible individuals [34]. QLF has also been claimed to be a sensitive enough method to be used in clinical trials comparing different preventive measures [35, 36]. In a clinical trial with 34 fifteen-year-old students with non-cavitated occlusal surfaces, QLF was more sensitive than meticulous visual inspection and yielded double the number of (presumed) carious sites [37]. QLF has

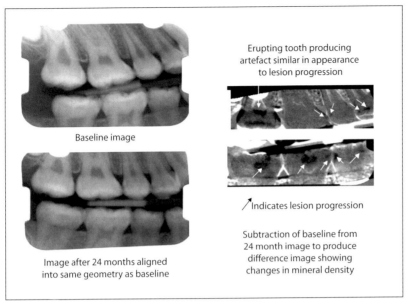

Fig. 4. Subtraction radiography requires 2 radiographs with exactly the same angulation.

also been tested in vivo in 44 eight-year-old children and was calculated to be able to assess lesion activity [38]. In a single-blind cluster randomized trial with 296 schoolchildren, QLF was used to calculate the remineralization capabilities of different fluoride-containing toothpastes on initial caries [39]. QLF is suitable for early lesion detection on smooth surfaces, although its validated performance in terms of sensitivity and specificity across the full range of caries predilection sites and the impact of surface staining are not yet established independently. However, its time-consuming image processing and analysis and its costs are the biggest obstacles for wide use in private dental practice. Concerning a wider use within this target group, a recently developed QLF-based tool for rapid, but not quantitative, caries detection might be promising [40].

Subtraction Radiography

Subtraction radiography is based on the principle that 2 radiographs taken with the same projection geometry are spatially and densitometrically aligned. They are then digitally subtracted to remove structural noise in the image. Following subtraction the contrast is stretched in the image. This process enhances any changes in the lesion between 2 points in time. This technique has been made a reality in the last decade, whereas earlier attempts had proved to be unsuccessful. It is clear that this subtraction process will not necessarily improve the *detection* of a lesion, but will only provide information on any changes occurring over time (fig. 4) and is therefore suitable for monitoring lesion behaviour. The system works well for approximal lesions and occlusal lesions in dentine. However, misalignment between images can produce edge effects at the boundary between enamel and dentine that can make interpretation of images difficult. Inclusion of a density reference in an image such as a step wedge can make the system quantitative.

Recently the utility of the method was investigated in a study which assessed the placement of fissure sealants on approximal lesions [41]. Radiographs were assessed independently, as pairs and using subtraction radiography after 18 months from placement of the sealant. For the independent radiograph assessment method, 10 and 26% progressed in the sealant and control groups, respectively ($p > 0.05$); with the paired radiograph method, the corresponding data were 22% in the test and 47% in the control groups ($p < 0.01$). By subtraction radiography, 44% of the test group and 84% of the control were judged to have progressed ($p < 0.001$). This study demonstrates the potential for the method, but further work is required to validate it. It is clear that by using digital technology there is great potential for improving the diagnostic yield from radiographs, and this is an area of research that is expected to grow as technology advances.

Electrical Caries Measurements

Over the last 6 decades, the relationship between the extent of caries in teeth and electrical resistance has been investigated. These investigations have focussed on the various parameters affecting electrical measurements of teeth, including porosity, surface area of the contact 'electrode', the thickness of enamel (and dentine) tissue, hydration of the enamel, temperature, ionic content (concentration) of the dental tissue fluids, as well as the maturation time of the tooth in the oral environment.

The validity of electrical caries detection methods was reviewed by Huysmans [42], as well as Longbottom and Huysmans [43], and subject to a systematic review by Bader et al. [44]. These mainly relate to the commercially available fixed-frequency ECM device (electronic caries monitor). The relatively few papers on this ECM published since those reviews indicate that only slight modifications are required to their conclusions.

The ECM device can be used in a 'site-specific' or 'surface-specific' mode, the latter involving a conducting medium used to cover the whole occlusal surface of a tooth – see table 1 for sensitivity and specificity values.

In vitro studies by Ellwood and Cortes [45] and Cortes et al. [46] indicated that the presence of stain is a confounder for ECM measurements and that different ECM cut-off values for enamel and dentine caries may be required for stained teeth.

The reproducibility of the device has been assessed and ranges from 0.53 to 0.92 for the site-specific and from 0.55 to 0.89 for the surface-specific method, but due to

Table 1. The range of values of sensitivity and specificity for ECM measurements for site- and surface-specific methods at the D_1 and D_3 thresholds for occlusal sites

	Site-specific		Surface-specific	
	sensitivity	specificity	sensitivity	specificity
D_1 (enamel)	0.70–0.92	0.78–1.00	0.61–0.65	0.73–0.86
D_3 (dentine)	0.39–0.97	0.56–0.98	0.68–0.78	0.76–0.90

the wide variations, Huysmans [42] cast doubt on its suitability for the longitudinal monitoring of lesion behaviour.

More recently, analysis by Huysmans et al. [47] has indicated that there may be a systematic error in the fixed-frequency ECM measurement technique, possibly attributable to inconsistent probe contact with the tooth surface. The authors suggested that a modification of the probe design may be necessary and a newer prototype device with such a modified probe design appears to reduce this systematic error [48].

Root Caries

A small number of studies have looked at the use of the fixed-frequency ECM for root caries detection. Wicht et al. [49] found a moderate relationship between ECM measurements and root caries lesion depth in an in vitro study. Baysan et al. [50], in vitro, and Petersson et al. [51], in vivo over 12 months, found that ECM measurements appeared capable of distinguishing between different severities of primary root caries lesions. Electrical measurements for caries detection have been investigated for several decades. The literature indicates that there is value in such measurements using fixed-frequency devices for dentine caries detection at occlusal sites. However, at present, there are limitations to these measurements, in particular in relation to the number of false-positive readings. This type of ECM may be used as an adjunct to clinical information and other detection methods. The use of multiple-frequency electrical caries measurement, using AC impedance spectroscopy, was reported with very encouraging in vitro results some time ago [52, 53]. The detection of caries and its extent, in terms of the order of magnitude differences between sound approximal surfaces, surfaces with initial lesions and surfaces with cavitation, was shown to be feasible [52, 53]. Although further development of a clinical device which can be used on other tooth surfaces has been reported in abstracts and a device is apparently now available to dentists in the UK, further published studies are required to assess the implementation of this technology further.

Conclusions

Four novel methods for non-invasive caries detection and – to a limited extent – caries monitoring are presented in this chapter. All methods presented have potential for wider use in the private clinical setting – the balance between enhancing the sensitivity of lesion detection and trading-off lower values for specificity must always be borne in mind and allowed for when making treatment decisions. All the methods presented require further research and further validation in well-designed clinical trials. In the future, these types of lesion detection aids could have useful applications in clinical practice as a complement to clinical visual lesion detection and as part of a personalized, comprehensive caries management system.

References

1. Lussi A, Imwinkelried S, Pitts N, Longbottom C, Reich E: Performance and reproducibility of a laser fluorescence system for detection of occlusal caries in vitro. Caries Res 1999;33:261–266.
2. König K, Flemming G, Hibst R: Laser-induced autofluorescence spectroscopy of dental caries. Cell Mol Biol (Noisy-le-Grand) 1998;44:1293–3000.
3. Buchalla W, Attin T, Niedmann Y, Niedmann PD: Porphyrins are the cause of red fluorescence of carious dentine: verified by gradient reversed-phase HPLC (abstract). Caries Res 2008;42:223.
4. Francescut P, Zimmerli B, Lussi A: Influence of different storage methods on laser fluorescence values: a two-year study. Caries Res 2006;40:181–185.
5. Ricketts D: The eyes have it: how good is Diagnodent at detecting caries? Evid Based Dent 2005;6:64–65.
6. Lussi A, Hibst R, Paulus R: Diagnodent: an optical method for caries detection. J Dent Res 2004;83(spec iss C):80–83.
7. Bader JD, Shugars DA: A systematic review of the performance of a laser fluorescence device for detecting caries. J Am Dent Assoc 2004;135:1413–1426.
8. Tranaeus S, Lindgren LE, Karlsson L, Angmar-Mansson B: In vivo validity and reliability of IR fluorescence measurements for caries detection and quantification. Swed Dent J 2004;28:173–182.
9. Lussi A, Hack A, Hug I, Heckenberger H, Megert B, Stich H: Detection of approximal caries with a new laser fluorescence device. Caries Res 2006;40:97–103.
10. Lussi A, Megert B, Longbottom C, Reich E, Francescut P: Clinical performance of a laser fluorescence device for detection of occlusal caries lesions. Eur J Oral Sci 2001;109:14–19.
11. Huth KC, Neuhaus KW, Gygax M, Bucher K, Crispin A, Paschos E, Hickel R, Lussi A: Clinical performance of a new laser fluorescence device for detection of occlusal caries lesions in permanent molars. J Dent 2008;36:1033–1040.
12. Bamzahim M, Aljehani A, Shi XQ: Clinical performance of Diagnodent in the detection of secondary carious lesions. Acta Odontol Scand 2005;63:26–30.
13. Bamzahim M, Shi XQ, Angmar-Mansson B: Secondary caries detection by Diagnodent and radiography: a comparative in vitro study. Acta Odontol Scand 2004;62:61–64.
14. Lennon AM, Buchalla W, Switalski L, Stookey GK: Residual caries detection using visible fluorescence. Caries Res 2002;36:315–319.
15. Aljehani A, Tranaeus S, Forsberg CM, Angmar-Mansson B, Shi XQ: In vitro quantification of white spot enamel lesions adjacent to fixed orthodontic appliances using quantitative light-induced fluorescence and Diagnodent. Acta Odontol Scand 2004; 62:313–318.
16. Aljehani A, Yousif MA, Angmar-Mansson B, Shi XQ: Longitudinal quantification of incipient carious lesions in postorthodontic patients using a fluorescence method. Eur J Oral Sci 2006;114:430–434.
17. Wicht MJ, Haak R, Stutzer H, Strohe D, Noack MJ: Intra- and interexaminer variability and validity of laser fluorescence and electrical resistance readings on root surface lesions. Caries Res 2002;36:241–248.
18. Takamori K, Hokari N, Okumura Y, Watanabe S: Detection of occlusal caries under sealants by use of a laser fluorescence system. J Clin Laser Med Surg 2001;19:267–271.

19 Diniz MB, Rodrigues JA, Hug I, Cordeiro RC, Lussi A: The Influence of pit and fissure sealants on infrared fluorescence measurements. Caries Res 2008;42:328–333.

20 Krause F, Braun A, Frentzen M: The possibility of detecting subgingival calculus by laser-fluorescence in vitro. Lasers Med Sci 2003;18:32–35.

21 Rodrigues J de A, Hug I, Diniz MB, Cordeiro RC, Lussi A: The influence of zero-value subtraction on the performance of two laser fluorescence devices for detecting occlusal caries in vitro. J Am Dent Assoc 2008;139:1105–1112.

22 Francescut P, Lussi A: Correlation between fissure discoloration, Diagnodent measurements, and caries depth: an in vitro study. Pediatr Dent 2003;25:559–564.

23 Lussi A, Reich E: The influence of toothpastes and prophylaxis pastes on fluorescence measurements for caries detection in vitro. Eur J Oral Sci 2005;113:141–144.

24 Lussi A, Zimmerli B, Hellwig E, Jaeggi T: Influence of the condition of the adjacent tooth surface on fluorescence measurements for the detection of approximal caries. Eur J Oral Sci 2006;114:478–482.

25 De Josselin de Jong E, Sundstrom F, Westerling H, Tranaeus S, ten Bosch JJ, Angmar-Mansson B: A new method for in vivo quantification of changes in initial enamel caries with laser fluorescence. Caries Res 1995;29:2–7.

26 Pitts NB, Longbottom C: The use of endoscopically viewed filtered fluorescence for the clinical diagnosis of carious lesions in dental enamel. Med Sci Res 1987;15:535–536.

27 Longbottom C, Pitts NB: An initial comparison between endoscopic and conventional methods of caries diagnosis. Quintessence Int 1990;21:531–540.

28 Al-Khateeb S, ten Cate JM, Angmar-Mansson B, de Josselin de Jong E, Sundstrom G, Exterkate RA, Oliveby A: Quantification of formation and remineralization of artificial enamel lesions with a new portable fluorescence device. Adv Dent Res 1997;11:502–506.

29 Kühnisch J, Ifland S, Tranaeus S, Angmar-Mansson B, Hickel R, Stösser L, Heinrich-Weltzien R: Establishing quantitative light-induced fluorescence cut-offs for the detection of occlusal dentine lesions. Eur J Oral Sci 2006;114:483–488.

30 Lagerweij M, van der Veen M, Ando M, Lukantsova L, Stookey G: The validity and repeatability of three light-induced fluorescence systems: an in vitro study. Caries Res 1999;33:220–226.

31 Tranaeus S, Shi XQ, Lindgren LE, Trollsas K, Angmar-Mansson B: In vivo repeatability and reproducibility of the quantitative light-induced fluorescence method. Caries Res 2002;36:3–9.

32 Van der Veen MH, Mattousch T, Boersma JG: Longitudinal development of caries lesions after orthodontic treatment evaluated by quantitative light-induced fluorescence. Am J Orthod Dentofacial Orthop 2007;131:223–228.

33 Mattousch TJ, van der Veen MH, Zentner A: Caries lesions after orthodontic treatment followed by quantitative light-induced fluorescence: a 2-year follow-up. Eur J Orthod 2007;29:294–298.

34 Al-Khateeb S, Forsberg CM, de Josselin de Jong E, Angmar-Mansson B: A longitudinal laser fluorescence study of white spot lesions in orthodontic patients. Am J Orthod Dentofacial Orthop 1998;113:595–602.

35 Tranaeus S, Al-Khateeb S, Bjorkman S, Twetman S, Angmar-Mansson B: Application of quantitative light-induced fluorescence to monitor incipient lesions in caries-active children: a comparative study of remineralisation by fluoride varnish and professional cleaning. Eur J Oral Sci 2001;109:71–75.

36 Karlsson L, Lindgren LE, Trollsas K, Angmar-Mansson B, Tranaeus S: Effect of supplementary amine fluoride gel in caries-active adolescents: a clinical QLF study. Acta Odontol Scand 2007;65:284–291.

37 Kühnisch J, Ifland S, Tranaeus S, Hickel R, Stosser L, Heinrich-Weltzien R: In vivo detection of non-cavitated caries lesions on occlusal surfaces by visual inspection and quantitative light-induced fluorescence. Acta Odontol Scand 2007;65:183–188.

38 Meller C, Heyduck C, Tranaeus S, Splieth C: A new in vivo method for measuring caries activity using quantitative light-induced fluorescence. Caries Res 2006;40:90–96.

39 Feng Y, Yin W, Hu D, Zhang YP, Ellwood RP, Pretty IA: Assessment of autofluorescence to detect the remineralization capabilities of sodium fluoride, monofluorophosphate and non-fluoride dentifrices: a single-blind cluster randomized trial. Caries Res 2007;41:358–364.

40 Van Daelen CJ, Smith PW, de Josselin de Jong E, Higham SM, van der Veen MH: A simple blue light to visualize caries by means of fluorescence. Caries Res 2008;42:223.

41 Martignon S, Ekstrand KR, Ellwood R: Efficacy of sealing proximal early active lesions: an 18-month clinical study evaluated by conventional and subtraction radiography. Caries Res 2006;40:382–388.

42 Huysmans MCDNJM: Electrical measurements for early caries detection; in Stookey GK (ed): Early Detection of Caries II. Proceedings of the 4th Annual Indiana Conference. Indianapolis, Indiana School of Dentistry, 2000, pp 123–142.

43 Longbottom C, Huysmans MCDNJM: Electrical measurements for use in clinical trials. J Dent Res 2004;83(spec iss C):76–79.

44 Bader JD, Shugars DA, Bonito AJ: A systematic review of the performance of methods for identifying carious lesions. J Public Health Dent 2002;62: 201–213.

45 Ellwood R, Cortes DF: In vitro assessment of methods of applying the electrical caries monitor for the detection of occlusal caries. Caries Res 2004;38:45–53.

46 Cortes DF, Ellwood R, Ekstrand KR: An in vitro comparison of a combined FOTI/visual examination of occlusal caries with other caries diagnostic methods and the effect of stain on their diagnostic performance. Caries Res 2003;37:8–16.

47 Huysmans MCDNJM, Kühnisch J, ten Bosch JJ: Reproducibility of electrical caries measurements: a technical problem? Caries Res 2005;39:403–410.

48 Kühnisch J, Heinrich-Weltzien R, Tabatabaie M, Stösser L, Huysmans MCDNJM: An in vitro comparison between two methods of electrical resistance measurement for occlusal caries detection. Caries Res 2006;40:104–111.

49 Wicht MJ, Haak R, Stutzer H, Strohe D, Noack MJ: Intra- and interexaminer variability and validity of laser fluorescence and electrical resistance readings on root surface lesions. Caries Res 2002;36:241–248.

50 Baysan A, Prinz JF, Lynch E: Clinical criteria used to detect primary root caries with electrical and mechanical measurements in vitro. Am J Dent 2004;7:94–99.

51 Petersson LG, Hakestam U, Baigi A, Lynch E. Remineralisation of primary root caries lesions using amine fluoride rinse and dentifrice twice a day. Am J Dent 2007;20:93–96.

52 Longbottom C, Huysmans MCDNJM, Pitts NB, Los P, Bruce PG: Detection of dental decay and its extent using AC impedance spectroscopy. Nat Med 1996;2: 235–237.

53 Huysmans MCDNJM, Longbottom C, Pitts NB, Los P, Bruce PG: Impedance spectroscopy of teeth with and without approximal carious lesions – an in vitro study. J Dent Res 1996;75:1871–1878.

Dr. Klaus W. Neuhaus
Department of Preventive, Restorative and Pediatric Dentistry, School of Dental Medicine
University of Bern, Freiburgstrasse 7
CH–3010 Bern (Switzerland)
Tel. +41 31 632 4974, Fax +41 31 632 9875, E-Mail Klaus.neuhaus@zmk.unibe.ch

Lesion Activity Assessment

K.R. Ekstrand[a] · D.T. Zero[b] · S. Martignon[d] · N.B. Pitts[c]

[a]Department of Cariology and Endodontics, University of Copenhagen, Copenhagen, Denmark; [b]Indiana University School of Dentistry, Indianapolis, Ind., USA; [c]Caries Research Unit UNICA, Dental Faculty, Universidad El Bosque, Bogotá, Colombia; [d]Dental Health Services and Research Unit, University of Dundee, Dundee, UK

Abstract

This chapter focusses on the probability of a caries lesion detected during a clinical examination being active (progressing) or arrested. Visual and tactile methods to assess primary coronal lesions and primary root lesions are considered. The evidence level is rated as low (R_w), as there are few studies with proper validation. The major problem is lack of an accepted clinical gold standard. Evidence from high-quality basic research and epidemiological, clinical and intervention studies is therefore discussed. High-quality basic research has mapped the patho-anatomical changes occurring in response to cariogenic plaque as well as lesion arrest. Based on this understanding, different clinical scoring systems have been developed to assess the severity/depth and activity of lesions. A recent system has been devised by the International Caries Detection and Assessment System Committee. The literature suggests that there is a fair agreement between visual/tactile external scripts of caries and the severity/depth of the lesion. The reproducibility of the different systems is, in general, substantial. No single clinical predictor is able to reliably assess activity. However, a combination of predictors increases the accuracy of lesion activity prediction for both primary coronal and root lesions. Three surrogate methods have been used for evaluating lesion activity (construct validity); all have disadvantages. If construct validity is accepted as a 'gold standard', it is possible to assess the activity of primary coronal and root lesions reliably and accurately at one examination by using the combined information obtained from a range of indicators – such as visual appearance, location of the lesion, tactile sensation during probing and gingival health.

Copyright © 2009 S. Karger AG, Basel

While *detecting* caries lesions is important, it only represents part of the caries diagnostic process. Optimally, the goal is to decide accurately and reliably (1) whether the observed condition is indeed a caries lesion and not something else (e.g. dental fluorosis), (2) assess its severity (depth and lateral extent) and finally (3) assess the activity status of the lesion [1]. If the caries lesion is then judged to be in a state of progression (an active caries lesion; fig. 1) (see also chapter by Longbottom et al., vol., pp. 209–216), and the relevant disease-promoting factors are anticipated to stay the same, some form of preventive/non-operative or operative treatment is needed. If, on

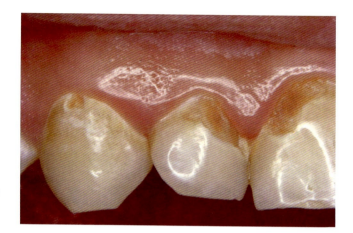

Fig. 1. Front teeth with caries which all dentists will state as active.

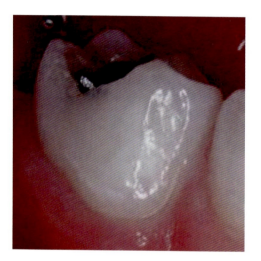

Fig. 2. A primary molar tooth with an arrested lesion on the buccal surface.

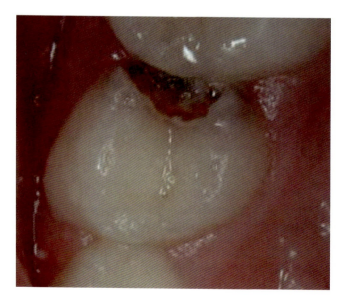

Fig. 3. A primary molar tooth with a cavitated lesion involving the dentine on the distal surface.

the other hand, the lesion is judged to be not progressing (an arrested lesion; fig. 2), and the relevant disease-promoting factors are anticipated to stay the same, no treatment is needed beyond background level care [1–3].

At least two diagnostic approaches have been considered. The first approach involves monitoring the lesion(s) over multiple clinical examinations for changes in their physical and/or optical properties. For this approach, International Caries Detection and Assessment System (ICDAS) severity scoring can be applied [4–6]. The second approach involves attempting to characterize caries lesion activity during a single clinical examination, in real time, in order to determine whether intervention is necessary and if so which treatment offers the best prognosis for the lesion/tooth/patient. For example, professional applied fluoride (fluoride varnish) to an approximal cavitated lesion, sensitive to sweets, on a 7-year-old child (fig. 3), is *not* the treatment offering the best prognosis for the tooth/patient; the lesion should rather be restored.

This chapter will focus on the likelihood or probability (or risk) that a caries lesion detected during a clinical examination is active (progressing) or is arrested, if the relevant disease-promoting factors stay the same. Primary coronal and root caries lesions detected by visual and visual-tactile methods will be considered.

In a recent report from Sweden [7], the evidence levels of different caries detection methods in detecting depth of the lesions were evaluated. In general, for the inclusion criteria specified, the result was weak in relation to the detection of lesions in enamel only, as distinct from lesions which had entered the dentine. Further, only a few studies were identified which included the aim of assessing caries activity in terms of specific lesions being active or arrested; however, none of these studies passed the inclusion criteria (e.g. lack of use of an accepted gold standard; <35 teeth included) set up by the committee. The authors of the present work repeated the literature search for caries activity studies, but came to the same conclusion as the Swedish report; thus, the evidence level of the studies concerning caries lesion activity assessment is placed low using the generally accepted evidence hierarchy (see e.g. SIGN Guidelines: www.sign.ac.uk) and is graded R_w according to the system used. Concerning the topic of lesion activity assessment during a single examination, we are therefore forced to deal with high-quality basic research, as well as with epidemiological, clinical studies and intervention studies, the two latter without optimal validation.

The chapter is structured as follows:
(a) patho-anatomical features of active and arrested lesions at the ultrastructural, histological and macroscopic/clinical levels;
(b) other indicators used in clinical caries lesion activity assessment;
(c) existing caries scoring systems with acceptable reliability and accuracy;
(d) discussion and conclusions;
(e) future research and implementation within the topic of lesion activity.

Patho-Anatomical Features of Active and Arrested Lesions

Dental caries (the disease) can be defined as 'the localized destruction of susceptible dental hard tissue by acidic by-products from bacterial fermentation of dietary carbohydrates' [see chapter by Longbottom et al., this vol., pp. 209–216]. The disease can also be considered as a diet-bacteria-induced slowly developing disease in the dental hard tissues [8]. The disease is caused by cariogenic plaque, in which some micro-organisms produce weak acids in particular lactic, as they metabolize dietary carbohydrates. The acids gradually dissolve the underlying mineral in the tooth, which may lead to irreversible structural changes (patho-anatomical changes) in the dental hard tissues. For the purpose of this chapter, the term 'patho-anatomical' changes should be understood as pathological changes from what is considered sound (healthy) tooth tissues, at the ultrastructural, histological and macroscopic/clinical level. When it comes to describing the patho-anatomical changes due to caries, the changes are normally described for both the external surface (at all three levels) and the subsurface tissue (most often at the histological level, due to limitations associated with tissue preparation).

Primary Coronal Caries

Enamel
Back in the 1980s, Thylstrup and his group [9–14] mapped the patho-anatomical changes in caries lesions on free smooth surfaces of premolar teeth scheduled for extraction because of orthodontic reasons. These lesions were deliberately provoked by initiating plaque stagnation under orthodontic bands, which were placed for 1, 2, 3 and 4 weeks [9, 10]. In a second study, 4-week-old lesions were created adjacent to orthodontic bands and subsequently the patho-anatomical changes were recorded after debonding over 1, 2 and 3 weeks [11–14].

Examination at the ultrastructural level showed that, in this aggressive clinical model, caries initiation begins with direct dissolution of the crystals in the surface enamel [14] rendering it softer [15]. Further cariogenic challenge leads to increased surface dissolution and preferential subsurface dissolution (at the ultrastructural and histological level), which changes the optical behaviour of the affected enamel. Eventually the dissolution results in the intercrystalline space/pore volume increasing to such an extent that incident light is refracted internally and back-scattered far more than in sound enamel [16]. This increase in back-scattering of the incident white light thereby produces the white appearance of the '*white-spot* lesion' – the enamel becomes slightly opaque (at the macroscopic/clinical level) and loses its surface luster (due to the decrease in reflection from the enamel surface and increased light-scattering). The term 'chalky' is perhaps the best word describing such lesions. Due to the direct dissolution of the crystals at the outer surface of enamel, the enamel lesion surface becomes slightly rough to tactile testing [14]. Analyses of subsurface enamel with histological techniques confirmed higher levels of porosity within white-spot lesions [14].

Thylstrup et al. [14] showed that mechanical removal of the cariogenic plaque from orthodontic-band-induced lesions after debracketing led to surface wear (abrasion), which resulted in removal of the most porous part of the surface enamel (at the ultrastructural level). The 'new' surface of the arrested lesion (at the macroscopic level) is therefore shiny (increased reflection and reduced light-scattering) and smooth to tactile probing, in contrast to the chalky, rough surface of the active lesion. The histological examination disclosed that the subsurface porosities deep into the arrested lesion were less than when the lesion was active, due to reprecipitation of minerals (remineralization) from the intercrystalline fluids. The relative contributions of wear and remineralization in arresting lesions which have not been induced with such an aggressive challenge (orthodontic-band-induced followed by professional and home based cleaning) are not well understood.

Other literature [for a review, see 17] indicates that the surface enamel of caries lesions is more fluoride rich and more permeable to dyes and radio-isotopes than sound enamel. Further, an active lesion should be more porous than an arrested lesion. Whether the level of porosity can be used reliably and accurately in differentiating between active and arrested lesions has, however, still to be evaluated.

Dentine

Dentine is a vital tissue, which reacts to any stimulus, including caries [18]. The reactions are dentinal sclerosis and reparative dentine formation, which will eventually change the colour of the dentine. This can be seen in elderly patients, where the teeth become yellowish. Sclerotic dentine due to caries can be observed histologically when the lesion has penetrated halfway through the enamel [19]. When acid from the bacterial deposits at the tooth surface penetrates the enamel and enters the sclerotic dentine, the now demineralized (sclerotic) dentine will change colour, becoming yellowish/brownish. Clinically, the changes can often be seen as a shadow on the surface (fig. 4a). The demineralization of the dentine results also in it becoming softer (fig. 4b).

Evidence of reparative dentine can be noted histologically when the lesion is deep in the enamel [20]. The quality of the reparative dentine is influenced by the caries progression rate: in cases with low progression rate, the reparative dentine consists of tubular dentine created by primary odontoblasts, and in cases with very fast progression rates, the odontoblasts may be harmed and other cells in the subodontoblastic region take part in the reparative dentine formation, resulting in an atubular form of reparative dentine. The colour of reparative dentine differs from sclerotic or demineralized dentine in that is has a greyish appearance.

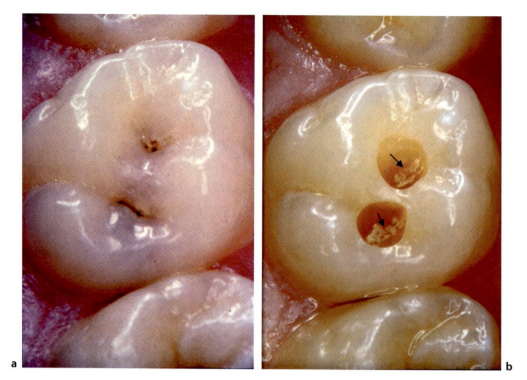

Fig. 4. a An upper molar with occlusal caries (shadow) which indicates that the dentine has been demineralized. **b** After removal of the enamel the dentine is light brown and soft to probing (arrows).

Primary Root Caries Lesions

Development of root caries requires recession of the gingiva. The aetiology of root caries is basically the same as that of coronal caries, although the pathogenesis is slightly different from primary coronal enamel and coronal dentine caries. For example, bacteria enter the dentinal tubules during very early stages of root caries development (when the cementum has been lost), in contrast to enamel caries where the bacteria enter enamel only after it has become highly demineralized, thus relatively late in lesion development. Further, root caries lesions tend to wrap around the whole cervical circumference of a tooth, but not to penetrate as deeply as coronal caries. Differences in the structure of the tissues, the directions of the prisms in enamel versus the orientation of the dentinal tubules and differences in access to saliva/gingival fluid are all important factors in explaining the differences in the pathogenesis of root caries lesions and enamel lesions. The dissolution of root dentine due to caries results in similar patho-anatomical changes as in coronal dentine (see above). As with enamel caries, the root caries dentine lesion is divided into a slightly demineralized surface lesion covering a more pronounced demineralized subsurface lesion [21].

Table 1. Visual and tactile characteristics for active and arrested lesions in enamel, coronal dentine and roots

	Visual	Tactile
Enamel		
Active	The lesion is whitish/yellowish; the lesion is chalky (lack of luster); the lesion can be cavitated or not	The lesion feels rough to probing; probing might or might not find a cavity
Arrested	The lesion is more yellowish/brownish than whitish; the lesion is more shiny than matte; the lesion can be cavitated or not	The lesion feels more smooth than rough; probing might or might not find a cavity
Coronal dentine		
Active	The lesion may manifest itself as a shadow below the intact but demineralized enamel; if a cavity extends into the dentine, the dentine appears yellowish/brownish	Dentine soft to probing
Arrested	The lesion may manifest itself as a shadow below the intact but demineralized enamel; if a cavity extends into the dentine, the dentine appears brownish	Harder than at the active lesion but not as hard as sound dentine
Root dentine		
Active	Yellowish/brownish	Soft/leathery
Arrested	Brownish/blackish	Harder but not as hard as sound root dentine

Table 1 summarizes clinically useful patho-anatomical changes characteristic of active and arrested lesions in enamel, coronal dentine and in root dentine.

Clinical Caries Assessment Indicators Other than the Patho-Anatomical Features in the Dental Hard Tissue

Presence of Plaque

As caries is a diet-bacteria-introduced disease, it is logical to use the presence of plaque as an indicator of the activity status of a lesion. However, controversy exists in the literature about the value of using plaque in judging activity of a caries lesion. Ekstrand et al. [22, 23] found for example weak correlations between the activity of occlusal as well as approximal lesions and the presence of plaque. Even when occlusal

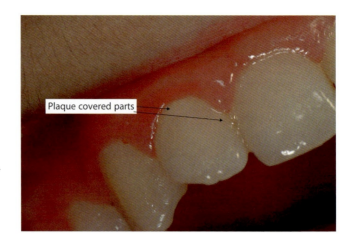

Fig. 5. Front teeth with proximal and gingival plaque. No lesions can be seen in the areas where the arrows are pointing.

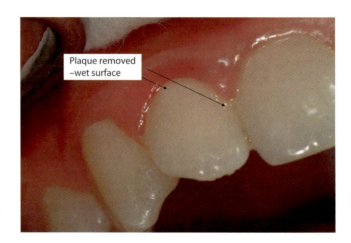

Fig. 6. Same front teeth as in figure 5; however, the plaque has been removed. Not sure if lesions (arrows) are present.

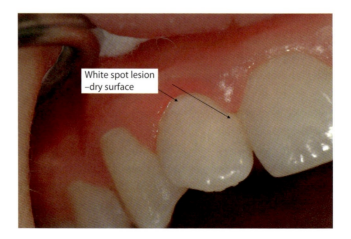

Fig. 7. Same front teeth as in figure 5 after drying, and now the initial lesions become visible (arrows).

plaque was divided by a colour method into cases with old plaque versus young plaque, the correlation did not increase [22]. On the other hand, Carvalho et al. [24] and Ekstrand et al. [25] found a significant correlation between plaque presence and active caries lesions on the occlusal surface of erupting permanent molars as well as on molars which had just reached full occlusion. One explanation why the presence of plaque is not a strong and consistent indicator for caries activity is that participants in investigations or regular patients in general have a better oral hygiene the day of an examination or dental visit than on other days.

Plaque Stagnation

In order to detect a caries lesion, in particular in its early stages, a tooth needs to be clean and dry [26, 27] (fig. 5–7). Thus, it is paradoxical that in order to initially identify the lesion, an examiner has to remove a potential indicator of activity, namely the plaque. A plaque stagnation area can be included as a surrogate. Thylstrup and Birkeland [28] stated that lesion progression can, under normal conditions, only occur in plaque stagnation areas. It is generally accepted that plaque stagnation areas are along the gingival margins, below (or above) approximal contact points and in the groove-fossa systems (pit and fissure systems). Ekstrand and Bjørndal [29] pointed to the fact that the micro-organisms in the deeper layer of narrow fissures are mostly non-vital and thus not cariogenic, while the entrance to the pits and fissures and the bottom as well as at the entrance to the more open fossa areas (compared to pits and fissures) harbour vital micro-organisms. As erupting occlusal surfaces accumulate significantly more plaque than when the same surfaces are in full occlusion [24, 25, 30], the entire occlusal surfaces, apart from the deepest parts of the pits and fissures, should be considered as a plaque stagnation area during the eruption period. After full occlusion has been established, only the entrance to the pits and fissures as well at the entrance and bottom part of the fossa areas are to be considered as stagnation areas with a cariogenic potential.

Gingival Status

It is generally accepted that the gingiva reacts via an inflammation process to regular plaque accumulation. Ekstrand et al. [23] found a substantial correlation between gingival inflammation and proximal caries and between gingival inflammation and lesion progression of approximal lesions in young adults. Lesion progression in that study was measured on radiographs taken at baseline and 1.5 years later.

Other Relevant Variables

There are also many 'determinants' that can influence the caries process by speeding up or slowing down the caries progression rate [31]. Saliva is a major determinant that slows down the caries progression rate by its cleansing of caries-promoting factors (oral bacteria and dietary carbohydrates), its dilution and buffering of plaque acids, its antimicrobial properties, and by providing inorganic and organic constituents that inhibit demineralization and promote remineralization and repair. Hyposalivation (<0.16 ml/min of unstimulated saliva) has been identified as a strong indicator that caries lesions will progress [32].

The age of the patient in relation to tooth eruption pattern should also be taken into consideration when evaluating the caries active status of a lesion. A white-spot lesion on a recently erupted tooth is more likely to be active than a white spot detected in an older individual long after a tooth has erupted. Caries susceptibility tends to decrease with age due to a posteruptive maturation process [33–35]. However, changes in caries-promoting factors and habits can overturn such a general pattern at the individual patient level. While the natural history of early caries lesions still requires further research, many white spots on older teeth are more likely to be scars from caries activity many years in the past.

Existing Caries Scoring Systems with Acceptable Reliability and Accuracy

Ismail [36] conducted a systematic review of visual and visuotactile scoring systems used for the detection and classification of dental caries from the 1950s up to 2000. A total of 29 studies were selected which met the inclusion criterion that there was a detailed description of the criteria used in the individual scoring system. All 29 systems focussed on caries detection in the tooth crown, while only 3 of the scoring systems also included criteria for the roots. In many cases, recording of caries adjacent to restorations (secondary caries) was included in the scoring systems. The degree of content validity (the extent to which the measurement incorporates the domain of the phenomenon under study) of the individual scoring systems was expressed by a summed score.

Using the framework of content validity as presented by Ismail [36], table 2 shows a total of 14 studies, dating from the early 60s up until today that included some kind of activity judgement in the scoring systems. Two of the scoring systems included suggestions which were untested [26, 37]. Two of the scoring systems were devised for root caries lesions only [39, 47].

The following parameters and scores were included to express the level of content validity (see explanation below table 2), levels for activity assessment (either 0, 1 or 2 points), levels of threshold (either 0, 1, 2 or 3 points), level of clarity of the scoring system (either 0 or 1 point), use of explorer (either 0 or 1 point), level of cleaning (either 0, 1 or 2 points) and level of drying of teeth (either 0, 1 or 2 points). The highest content validity (11 points) was seen in the studies by Fejerskov et al. [39] and Ekstrand et al. [6, 22, 46, 47], primarily because these scoring systems used more than 2 thresholds, professional cleaning and air-drying of teeth.

Table 2 also shows the level of reliability of the scoring systems expressed by κ in 10 of the 14 individual studies. The reliability seems to be substantial to excellent in all the studies, apart from the study by Ekstrand et al. [46], which focussed on very minute caries changes, where the reliability was poor (see explanation later).

Finally, only two groups of authors (5 studies in table 2) have validated the accuracy of the scoring systems in terms of construct validity (see definition later). The following paragraph will describe these 5 studies in detail.

In vitro Studies Dealing with Reliability (Reproducibility) and Accuracy

Based on the findings of Thylstup and his group (see above), Ekstrand et al. [48] devised a scoring system initially to detect occlusal lesions and predict their depth and later also to assess lesion activity [22]. Table 3 presents the visual criteria to detect depth (A) and the criteria characterizing the histological depth (B). When tested it was found that the scoring system could predict the depth of the lesion fairly well, as the correlation coefficients ranged from substantial to strong (r_s or r >0.72) [22, 48–51]. Further, in a number of studies the intra-examiner reliability ranged from substantial to excellent, and the interexaminer reliability ranged from moderate to substantial [48, 49, 51].

Concerning activity assessment, a study was initiated using 35 third molars scheduled for extraction, because it was possible to histologically validate the activity status of the lesion [22]. Just before extraction, the teeth were visually examined using the scoring system in table 3 (C). The original scores 1 and 2 (table 3, column A) with no divisions between white or brown spots was in the modified (activity) scoring system (table 3, column C) subdivided into scores 1 and 1a and 2 and 2a. Scores 1 and 2 were devoted to white-spot lesions and 1a and 2a to brown-spot lesions. This division was made because studies by Thylstrup and his group found (see above) that detection of a white-spot lesion indicated lesion progression, while a brown-spot lesion indicated that the lesion was arrested. After extraction and sectioning of the teeth, methyl red dye was applied to the exposed face of ground sections allowing diffusion through the lesions to establish whether the pH in the lesion was above or below 5.5 (the validation criteria). Methyl red changes colour at a pH around 5.5 [52], which is at the level where hydroxyapatite dissolves [53, 54]. By means of the methyl red, 22 of the 35 lesions were considered to be active (became red after application of methyl red = pH below 5.5, fig. 8a–c), the remaining 13 lesions as arrested (fig. 9a–c). When the visual scores 1, 2, 3 and 4 were used as indicators for active lesions

Table 2. Content validity, reliability and construct validity in 14 studies dealing with caries activity assessment

Scoring system	Year and country	Disease process	Thresholds	Subjectivity	Use of explorer	Cleaning of teeth	Drying of teeth	Total score	Reliability	Accuracy (construct validity)
Møller [26]	1966, Denmark	1	2	1	1	2	2	9	no	no
Howat [37]	1981, UK (visual-tactile method)	1	2	1	1	1	2	8	no	no
Pitts and Fyffe [38]	1988, HK	0	2	1	0	1	2	6	intra-examiner agreement: $D_3 = 0.789$, $D_2 = 0.818$, $D_1 = 0.795$	no
Fejerskov et al. [39]	1991, Denmark	2	3	1	1	2	2	11	intra-examiner agreement: $\kappa = 0.88$	no
Ismail et al. [40]	1992, Canada	2	3	1	1	1	1	9	2 examiners, intra- and interexaminer agreement: $\kappa > 0.8$	no
Rosen et al. [41]	1996, Sweden (crown and roots)	2	2	1	1	2	0	8	3 examiners, intra-examiner agreement: 0.47–0.61, interexaminer agreement: 0.29–0.51	no
Amarante et al. [42]	1998, Norway (coronal, secondary caries)	0	2	1	1	2	2	8	5 examiners, intra-examiner agreement: 0.92–0.95, interexaminer agreement: 0.80–0.93	no
Ekstrand et al. [22]	1998, Denmark	2	3	1	0	2	2	10	refer back to Ekstrand et al. [48]; 3 examiners, intra-examiner agreement: 0.73–0.89, interexaminer agreement: 0.54–0.69	methyl red polarized light examination; correlation coefficient: 0.88

Table 2. Continued

Scoring system	Year and country	Disease process	Thresholds	Subjectivity	Use of explorer	Cleaning of teeth	Drying of teeth	Total score	Reliability	Accuracy (construct validity)
Nyvad et al. [43]	1999, Lithuania	2	3	1	1	1	1	9	2 examiners. intra-examiner agreement: 0.74–0.85, interexaminer agreement: 0.78–0.80	no
Fyffe et al. [44]	2000, UK	2	2	1	1	1	2	9	inter-examiner agreement: novice 0.47–0.63, experienced 0.52–0.67	no
Nyvad et al. [45]	2003, Lithuania	2	3	1	1	1	1	9	Refer back to Nyvad et al. [43]	fluoride, for relative risk, see table 5
Ekstrand et al. [46]	2005, Denmark	2	3	1	1	2	2	11	3 examiner intra-examiner agreement: 0.24–0.66, interexaminer agreement: –0.08–0.26	impression material, perfect agreement 83%
Ekstrand et al. [6]	2007, Denmark	2	3	1	1	2	2	11	1 examiner, intra-examiner agreement: visual 0.87, plaque stagnation 0.63, tactile 0.63	impression material, sensitivity: 84%, specificity: 79%
Ekstrand et al. [47]	2008, Denmark	2	3	1	1	2	2	11	1 examiner, intra-examiner agreement: 0.86	impression material, sensitivity: 86%, specificity: 81%

Disease process: 0 = measure arrested and active lesions together; 1 = measure arrested and active lesions separately; 2 = measure arrested and active lesions separately at least of 2 different stages.
Thresholds: 0 = only cavitated lesion; 1 = non-cavitated and cavitated lesion; 2 = as 1 but with different stages of cavitated lesions; 3 = as 2 but with different stages of non-cavitated lesions also. Subjectivity: 0 = criteria contain vague terms that may increase examiner subjectivity; 1 = criteria clearly define the terms used to measure the caries process. Probe or explorer: 0 = no use; 1 = use. Cleaning teeth: 0 = no cleaning; 1 = the patients clean themselves; 2 = professional cleaning. Drying teeth/lesion: 0 = no drying; 1 = drying the mouth with e.g. cotton rolls; 2 = drying with air. Total score between 0 and 11. Reliability expressed by κ values. Accuracy expressed by sensitivity/specificity or related terms.

Table 3. Scores and criteria used by Ekstrand et al. [22] to assess coronal caries lesions on occlusal surfaces on permanent teeth

(A) Detection criteria		(B) Histological criteria		(C) Activity criteria	
code	criteria	code	criteria	code	criteria
0	No or slight change in enamel translucency after prolonged air-drying (>5 s)	0	No enamel demineralization or narrow surface zone of opacity (edge phenomenon)	0	No or slight change in enamel translucency after prolonged air-drying (>5 s)
1	Opacity or discolouration hardly visible on the wet surface, but distinctly visible after air-drying	1	Enamel demineralization limited to outer 50% of the enamel layer	1	Opacity (white) hardly visible on the wet surface, but distinctly visible after air-drying
				1a	Opacity (brown) hardly visible on the wet surface, but distinctly visible after air-drying
2	Opacity or discolouration distinctly visible without air-drying	2	Demineralization involving between 50% of the enamel and one third of the dentine	2	Opacity (white) distinctly visible without air-drying
				2a	Opacity (brown) distinctly visible without air-drying
3	Localized enamel breakdown in opaque or discoloured enamel and/or greyish discolouration from the underlying dentine	3	Demineralization involving the middle third of dentine	3	Localized enamel breakdown in opaque or discoloured enamel and/or greyish discolouration from the underlying dentine
4	Cavitation in opaque or discoloured enamel exposing the dentine	4	Demineralization involving the inner third of the dentine	4	Cavitation in opaque or discoloured enamel exposing the dentine

and scores 0, 1a and 2a as indications for sound or inactive lesions (table 3, column C), a strong and significant association was observed with the histological validation (contingency coefficient C = 0.88, p < 0.001 [22]). Subsequent analysis disclosed that in 9 of the 35 (26%) cases an incorrect clinical diagnosis was made compared to the histological assessment.

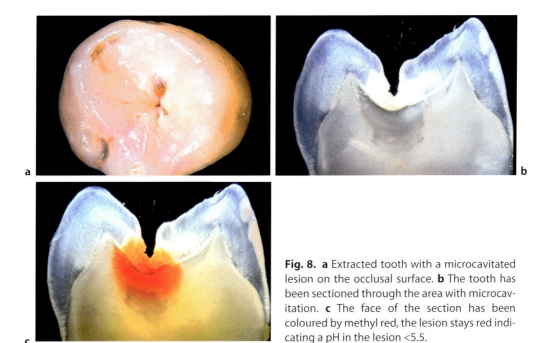

Fig. 8. a Extracted tooth with a microcavitated lesion on the occlusal surface. **b** The tooth has been sectioned through the area with microcavitation. **c** The face of the section has been coloured by methyl red, the lesion stays red indicating a pH in the lesion <5.5.

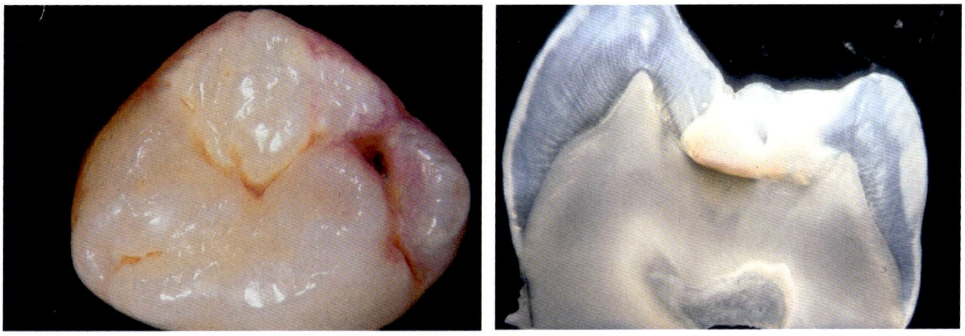

Fig. 9. a Extracted tooth with brown-spot lesions in the distal part of the occlusal surface. **b** The tooth has been sectioned through the area with the brown spot. **c** The face of the section has been coloured by methyl red, the lesion stayed yellowish indicating a pH in the lesion >5.5.

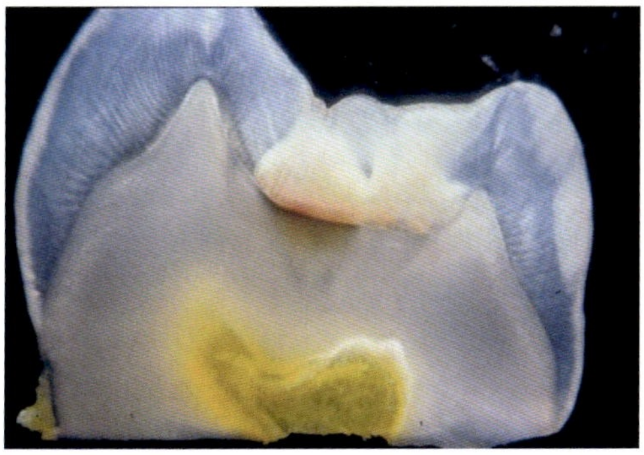

Lesion Activity Assessment

Table 4. Scores and categories used by Nyvad et al. [43] to assess coronal caries lesions

Score	Category
0	sound
1	active caries (intact surface)
2	active caries (surface discontinuity)
3	active caries (cavity)
4	inactive caries (intact surface)
5	inactive caries (surface discontinuity)
6	inactive caries (cavity)
7	filling (sound)
8	filling + active caries
9	filling + inactive caries

Table 5. The relative risk that a fluoride-exposed surface versus a non-fluoride-exposed surface undergoes caries lesion transition between baseline and a 3-year follow-up [45]

Baseline findings	Relative risk	Transition after 3 years
Sound	0.99	inactive lesions
Sound	0.72	active lesions
Sound	0.77	cavitated lesions
Inactive non-cavitated	0.35	active lesions
Inactive non-cavitated	0.72	cavitated lesions
Active non-cavitated	1.60	sound surfaces
Active non-cavitated	1.28	inactive lesions
Active non-cavitated	0.60	cavitated lesion
Unerupted	1.08	sound
Unerupted	0.47	active lesion
Unerupted	0.51	cavitation

A value of 1 indicates equal risk for transition in the two groups. A value lower than 1 means that the risk is higher in the control group than in the test group and vice versa.

Clinical Studies Dealing with Reliability (Reproducibility) and Accuracy

As indicated in table 4, the Nyvad system is a combined visuotactile caries diagnostic system involving 10 categories/scores. The criteria were based on the patho-anatomical changes occurring during the caries process described, amongst others, by Thylstrup and his group (see above). The reproducibility of the scoring system was first tested in a suboptimal clinical setting in Kaunas, Lithuania [43]. Intra-examiner κ values ranged between 0.74 and 0.85 and interexaminer ones between 0.78 and 0.80. The major problem, according to the authors, was consistency when differentiating sound sites from non-cavitated lesions (active as well as inactive).

Determination of the accuracy of the Nyvad criteria in assessing caries lesion activity was subsequently reported [45] after a 3-year longitudinal study. This study involved daily supervised brushing with a fluoride dentifrice by children in the test group (n = 193 children) versus a control group where the childrens' brushing was unsupervised (n = 80 children). The study evaluated the relative risk of transitions (progression or regression) of lesions from the test group versus the control group. The authors found, for example, that the sound and unerupted surfaces in the test group had a lower relative risk of progressing to active non-cavitated or cavitated lesions compared to similar baseline-scored surfaces of children in the control group (table 5). Furthermore, the baseline-scored active non-cavitated lesions in the test group had a higher chance of becoming sound or inactive than did the corresponding baseline lesions in the control group (table 5). Thus, the authors stated that the activity criteria (table 4) were capable of reflecting their hypothesized fluoride effect (inhibition of lesion progression/enhancing lesion regression) and thus established construct validity (see definition later). It is important to mention that a number of lesions did not follow the hypothesized effect of fluoride; thus in the control group, for example, 22% of the baseline-scored active non-cavitated lesions were scored as arrested non-cavitated lesions after 3 years and 22% had regressed to sound. Hence, roughly every second active non-cavitated lesion in the control group did not follow the predicted direction. Clinically this is not necessarily a problem as many early active lesions will arrest naturally [55, 56], but from a validation point of view it is problematic.

The Nyvad criteria used specific patho-anatomical changes to differentiate active from arrested lesions. Lack of luster and the presence of roughness were designated as indicating that the lesion was active, whereas arrested lesions were shiny and smooth. As mentioned above, an acceptable level of reproducibility was obtained by the Nyvad system, which may be related to the very thorough (several weeks) training before the start of the study.

Ekstrand et al. [46] investigated whether general dentists were able to determine reliably such subtle visual and tactile differences as lack of luster versus shiny aspect and roughness versus smoothness between active and inactive enamel lesions based on a single examination. Ten children with at least 4 non-cavitated active lesions (40 lesions) were included in the study. Full upper and lower impressions were taken, using the impression-based diagnostic material suggested by Schmid et al. [57] (Clinpro, 3M-ESPE). This was carried out to confirm the metabolic activity in terms of detecting lactic acid of any plaque overlying the selected lesions. A dark blue area on the impression surface indicates lactic acid production and a metabolically active plaque covering the corresponding lesion (potentially active lesion) on the tooth. Where no blue colour change was seen, the lesion was characterized as an arrested

Table 6. Scores and criteria used by Ekstrand et. [46] to assess coronal caries lesions on primary as well as permanent teeth

	Teeth	Visual scoring								Probing		
		nothing	dull white	dull white discoloured	dull discoloured	white glossy	white glossy discoloured	discoloured glossy	Σ	rough	smooth	Σ
Ex. 1	A	5	6	1	3	14	1	0	30	3	27	30
	B	1	3	1	1	3	0	1	10	2	8	10
Ex. 2	A	7	12	4	1	5	0	1	30	14	16	30
	B	0	3	3	0	3	0	1	10	4	6	10
Ex. 3	A	5	7	2	3	11	2	3	30	9	21	30
	B	0	2	4	1	3	0	0	10	2	8	10

Ex. = Examiner; A = professionally cleaned teeth, 30 lesions to be scored visually and the same 30 lesions to be scored by probing; B = control teeth, 10 lesions to be scored visually and the same 10 lesions to be scored by probing.

lesion. In 37 cases of the 40 selected (active) lesions, there was a corresponding colour change in the impression material (93% agreement). Three of the 4 lesions in each individual were then randomly selected to be professionally cleaned 5 days a week for 3–4 consecutive weeks. The fourth lesion was not cleaned professionally. Thus, a total of 30 lesions, or 3 lesions per subject, were expected to arrest during the study period while 10 lesions (1 per subject) were anticipated to continue to be active.

Table 6 shows the visual and tactile scorings used in the study and the distribution of the assessments related to score for the professionally cleaned lesions (A) and control lesions (B). Three very experienced dentists took part in the study, and they received a 10-min instruction in the scoring system. The results were poor in terms of accuracy (finding which lesions where active or arrested). Of the 30 lesions that were professionally cleaned and likely to be inactive (specificity), only between 50 and 73% were correctly judged by the dentists to be inactive. Of the 10 control teeth with active lesions (sensitivity) only 20–50% were correctly judged by the dentists as being active. The intra-examiner reproducibility for (a) visual, (b) tactile and (c) lesion activity was fair to moderate: (a) κ = 0.35–0.52, perfect agreement 50–70%; (b) κ = 0.24–0.66, perfect agreement 75–80%; (c) κ = 0.31–0.54, perfect agreement 50–70%. The interexaminer reproducibility was in general poor: (a) κ = 0.06–0.25, perfect agreement 32–43%; (b) κ = –0.08 to 0.26, perfect agreement 45–73%; (c) κ = 0.06–0.16, perfect agreement 43–45%. A possible limitation of this study is that a 30-day period of forced oral hygiene was insufficient to alter the clinical presentation of the lesions, the training time was too short and the study took part in a school and not in a clinical setting.

Based on the experience from the above study, Ekstrand et al. [6] suggested the use of 3 other clinical parameters, but used in combination, to assess the activity of

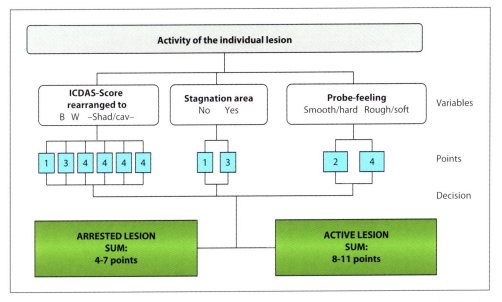

Fig. 10. Process of deciding whether a lesion (e.g. those seen in fig. 7) is arrested or active. On the first level, the 3 variables are scored: the ICDAS codes are rearranged into brown (B), white (W) and shadowed/cavitated (shad./cav.) lesions, whether the lesion is located in a plaque stagnation area or not and whether the lesion is smooth/hard or rough/soft. The second level is allocating points or a score. The third level shows the decision. If there are between 4 and 7 points, the lesion is likely arrested; if there are more than 7 points, the lesion is likely active.

coronal primary caries lesions. The first parameter was the visual signs of caries, and for this the lesions were initially classified using the ICDAS-II system and then rearranged in 3 groups: if the lesion was brown, white or microcavitated/shadowed/frank cavitation. The second parameter was lesion location in relation to plaque stagnation, i.e. whether or not the lesion was located in a plaque stagnation area. Finally, the third parameter was if the lesion was rough/soft or smooth/hard to probing.

The reliability (table 2) and accuracy of the scoring system was assessed in a study conducted in Bogota, Colombia, involving 36 children aged 5–11 years with 123 lesions. The accuracy of the variables and their subdivisions were evaluated (validated), by the responses from the Clinpro impressions taken a week after the clinical assessment. Initially, the study mapped the relative weight that each of the subdivisions within the 3 variables had in the activity assessment. Thus, it was observed that in 15% of the cases where the lesion was scored as brown there was a positive response (lactic acid) in the impression material; in contrast, in 85% of the brown-spot lesions there were no responses. The predictive weight of a brown-spot lesion was allocated 1 point (fig. 10). In the case where the lesion was white or cavitated, the positive response from the impression material was 45 and 75%, respectively – the predictive weight of these categories was allocated 3 and 4 points. Concerning

Table 7. Scores and criteria used by Ekstrand et al. [47] to assess root caries lesions on permanent teeth

Criteria	Points
Texture of the lesion when gently probed	
Hard	0
Leathery	1
Soft	3
Contour of the surface	
No cavitation or the surroundings of the cavity smooth to probing	1
Cavity with irregular border	2
Distance from the lesion to the gingival margin	
≥1 mm	1
<1 mm	2
Colour of the lesion	
Dark brown/black	1
Light brown/yellowish	2

A total score of 3–5 means lesion arrested, a total score of 6–9 indicates an active lesion.

the predictive value of the other 2 parameters, namely plaque stagnation and tactile perception, the calculations of the number of cases related to the positive response in the impression material resulted in a score of 1 for non-plaque stagnation area and 3 for the plaque stagnation, and 2 for smooth/hard and 4 for rough/soft, respectively (fig. 10). The study found that a cumulative sum of more than 7 points had the highest accuracy expressed by means of sensitivity (84%) and specificity (79%), using the Clinpro response for validation (fig. 10). The reliability of each of the 3 parameters was substantial to excellent. It is important to underline that the purpose of the scoring system was that the examiner should score, but not state if the lesion was active or arrested; the categorization of the latter was determined by the computation of the 3 component scores.

Activity Assessment of Root Caries Lesions

Fejerskov et al. [39] were among the first who suggested including activity assessment of root caries lesions in epidemiological surveys. Prior to this, Nyvad and Fejerskov [58] described that active root caries lesions were found next to the gingival margin, whereas arrested lesions were located some distance from the gingival margin. The authors also described the clinical changes that occurred with presumably active root caries lesions after meticulous toothbrushing with a fluoride toothpaste during a 2- to 6-month period. They observed that the active lesions, which were soft, greasy and yellowish at baseline, changed to leathery or hard, darkly discoloured tissue. The findings of Lynch and Beighton [59] agreed in principle with these observations based on their laboratory evidence using microbiological indicators for lesion activity, which showed that 'soft' or 'leathery' lesions on root surfaces are more heavily infected with bacteria than are 'hard' root surfaces. There is a general consensus, that colour of the root caries lesion is a poor predictor when it comes to activity assessment [59].

Based on the above, Ekstrand et al. [47] suggested 4 variables (table 7) to be used in combination to assess activity of root caries lesions. The points (1–3) attributed to the subdivisions for each variable were summed to give a total score, and a total score of 3–5 points characterized lesions as arrested and one of 6–9 as active. The accuracy of the devised scoring system was evaluated by means of Clinpro impression material (see above). The sensitivity and specificity values were 86 and 81%, respectively. Intrareproducibility expressed as perfect agreement on percentage of the individual parameters was: texture 82%, contour 92%, location 98% and colour 79%. As with the system for coronal lesions [6], the system is designed so that the examiner should score parameters, but not directly assess whether the lesion is active or arrested; that designation is determined by the computation.

Discussion and Conclusions

Özer and Thylstrup [60] proposed that caries adjacent to restorations is in fact primary caries next to restorations and should theoretically show similar features to primary caries in relation to lesion activity assessment. However, as yet, there are no reports of clinical studies and only sparse information from in vitro studies to support their contention. We decided, therefore, only to address activity assessment for primary caries on the crown and roots with the full knowledge that there is not the highest evidence level even for them. The major problem, which is difficult to address in study design, is to find a gold standard which can reliably differentiate between active and arrested lesions. Based on Wulff [61], Wenzel and Hintze [62] stated that any robust gold standard must fulfil three criteria: (1) it should be established by a method that is itself precise, i.e. reproducible (e.g. colour changes), (2) it should reflect the criteria which define the disease (e.g. lactic acid, patho-anatomical changes) and (3) it should be established independently of the diagnostic method under evaluation (if visual and tactile examination, then radiographs, impression material etc. could be used to compare with it).

Irrespective of the fact that there is a lack of studies evaluating the accuracy of assessing activity of caries lesions, a number of authors have devised caries scoring systems for a number of purposes, such as epidemiological, clinical studies and clinical intervention studies. The majority of these studies have devised caries recording systems based on the visually discernible patho-anatomical changes which occur as caries moves from its initial stage to its more profound stages. Therefore, this chapter initially describes the most relevant patho-anatomical changes due to caries in enamel and dentine. Actually, there is general consensus regarding these clinically apparent relevant patho-anatomical changes. The problem arises when it comes to testing the reproducibility of identifying particular characteristics, because some of them, e.g. dullness/lack of luster and shiny appearance, are very subtle changes and involve a relatively high degree of subjectivity.

Construct Validity

Within the last 10 years, first Ekstrand et al. [22], Nyvad et al. [45], then again Ekstrand et al. [6, 46, 47] have tried to overcome the problem of the lack of a gold standard in evaluating the accuracy of diagnostic methods for activity by using construct validity. According to Last [63], construct validity is 'the extent to which the measurement corresponds to theoretical concepts (constructs) concerning the phenomenon under study'. For example, on a theoretical basis, the phenomenon of gradual softening of enamel and dentine due to demineralization in an active lesion is amenable to testing for construct validity, since it can be assessed during an examination (fig. 4b) as well as longitudinally between two or more examinations using probing. Ekstrand and his group have used two different approaches for assessing caries lesion activity: (1) methyl red indicating a pH lower than 5.5 in the lesion [22] and (2) colour changes in impression material as evidence of lactic acid production in the overlying plaque [6, 46, 47] as a form of construct validity. Nyvad et al. [45] used the well-established therapeutic effects of fluoride in this regard. All three methods have disadvantages and can only be said to function as *surrogates* for whether the lesion is active or arrested per se.

Methyl red is a pH indicator which changes colour from yellow to red, when the pH falls below 5.5 [52]. A pH below 5.5 is considered to be the critical level for dissolution of hydroxyapatite [54]. Furthermore, measurements of pH in dentine lesions showed that in active dentine lesions the pH varied from 4.0 to 5.4, with an average of 4.9, contrasting to a mean pH of 5.7 (5.5–6.9) in inactive dentine lesions [64]. Thus, active lesions should be red after methyl red treatment (fig. 8) and arrested lesions yellowish (fig. 9). As such, methyl red seems promising to use for construct validity – actually it is close to fulfilling all 3 criteria to be a robust gold standard. However, methyl red cannot be used clinically, so it is only possible to extrapolate from laboratory research to clinical studies.

Concerning fluoride, it is well established and accepted that fluoride reduces the progression rate of caries lesions [65]. This view includes the logic that fluoride can reduce the progression rate of both very small, preclinical, 'invisible' lesions to an extent that it will take longer before they become clinically visible, as well as reducing

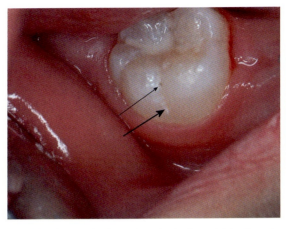
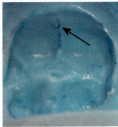

Fig. 11. Photo of a buccal caries lesion which after cleaning has been scored 11 points (visually microcavitated = 3 points; plaque stagnation area = 3 points and rough to probing = 4 points). After a week, the patient was asked to come to the clinic again; he was asked to brush his teeth, and an impression was taken with the Clinpro impression material. There is a signal (arrow) exactly corresponding to the location of the buccal lesion.

the progression rate of visible non-cavitated lesions so it takes a longer time before they will cavitate if the cariogenic challenge continues. Other authors suggest that fluoride can actually inhibit – i.e. stop – caries progression [45]. If the former theory is correct, it is not valid to use the effect of fluoride as a form of construct validity, as a lesion cannot be *arrest*ed by fluoride if it only *reduces* the caries progression rate. If the latter theory is correct, it may be possible to use the effect of fluoride as a form of construct validity. In the present authors' opinion, it is fair to state that the Nyvad scoring system has predictive value and is therefore interesting for the purpose of this chapter. The content validity is however only moderate (table 2), mainly because the system does not clean and dry the individual lesions.

In the clinical studies performed by Ekstrand et al. [6, 46, 47], the impression material Clinpro Caries Diagnosis Full Arch Lactic Acid Locator was used as a form of construct validity, as it has been shown to measure lactic acid production in plaque [57]. It is important to highlight that lactic acid is the principal acid in the demineralization process [66] – indeed it would be difficult for caries to develop in vivo without the presence of lactic acid. However, the presence of lactic acid per se does not mean that dissolution will always occur. The impression material consists of a powder which is mixed with an activator in order to induce setting. It also contains a sugar solution, which the micro-organisms metabolize during the 3 min it takes for the material to set. Fermentation of sugar and production of lactic acid by oral micro-organisms is almost immediate [66], and the result is an increasing fraction of lactic acid production [66]. The lactic acid initiates an indicator reaction within the impression material, turning it blue where the concentration of lactic acid is >4 mM (fig. 11).

Table 8. Data from impression with Clinpro in terms of signal/no signal and if the pH measured by a pH-meter was ≤5.5 or >5.5 [47]

	pH ≤5.5	pH >5.5	Total
No signal	1	12	13
Signal	26	6	32
	27	18	45
	sensitivity 26/27 = 0.96	specificity 12/18 = 0.67	

In the study by Ekstrand et al. [6] the Clinpro material was validated in terms of its accuracy in identifying lesions which were measured with a pH-meter to have a pH ≤5.5, discriminating them from lesions which had a pH >5.5. Table 7 shows the result from that study which included 9 persons, each having 3 dentine specimens inserted into their partial denture for a period of 6 weeks. Each of the 3 specimens received different treatment modalities during the 6-week period. Twice during the 6-week period, the pH was measured at the surface of the dentine specimens, and impressions were taken with Clinpro material. It appears from table 8 that the accuracy of the material was substantial in terms of sensitivity and specificity (combined 1.63) the magnitude of which is regarded as acceptable for a diagnostic test [67]. A more powerful scientific proof of the Clinpro material to assess lesion activity would be if multiple impressions are taken over a period of time, for example a week, before the clinical examination and every week during a month after the examination. At the moment, the Clinpro impression material is the validation method which comes closest to fulfilling the 3 criteria to be a robust gold standard: (a) the colour changes in the impression material give evidence of the presence of lactic acid which is easy to see (fig. 11), thus high reproducibility is possible; (b) it measures lactic acid, which is the most important acid in cariogenic plaque, and (c) the signal in the impression material is independent of the visual and tactile methods covered in this chapter. However, longitudinal studies are still required to determine if Clinpro is capable of predicting whether lesions designated as being active progress to cavitation and lesions designated as inactive stay arrested or become undetectable.

From the above, it can be stated that caries activity assessment based on a single examination is about likelihoods, probability or risk. No single category or clinical parameter appears sufficient for assessment of whether a lesion is active or arrested. Even in apparently obvious cases (fig. 1), at least 3 categories will indicate that the lesions on the incisors and the canine are active, considered in the present chapter as 'the lesions which will progress if the relevant disease-promoting factors are not changed': (1) the major part of the lesions are cavitated with irregular borders, (2) the dentine is soft and (3) the lesions are next to the gingival margin (plaque stagnation area), which by the way is also inflamed.

Based on the literature, the following can be concluded about lesion activity assessment, related to one single examination (i.e. at one point in time):

(1) a reliable current and accurate gold standard for caries activity assessment, based on one examination, is not available;
(2) the studies that have been undertaken thus far to investigate different systems for assessing caries activity are therefore not placed very high in the evidence hierarchy (R_w);
(3) if construct validity is accepted as a 'gold standard', this review indicates that it is possible to assess the activity of primary coronal and root caries lesions reliably and accurately at one examination by using the combined information obtained from a range of indicators, such as visual appearance of the lesion, location of the lesion, tactile sensation during probing and gingival health.

Future Research and Implementation with the Topic of Lesion Activity

Priorities for *future research* are:
- studies designed to provide a better understanding of the natural history of caries lesions, particularly the 'early' primary lesion, as well as of caries associated with restorations;
- development of objective tools to characterize the caries activity of (early) lesions both in real time and monitoring over time;
- exploration of the role of surface porosity in the caries process and its potential use in activity assessment;
- development of a widely accepted gold standard for caries lesion activity.

Priorities for the *implementation* of existing research are generally around overcoming the barriers in some geographic locations associated with:
- the lack of familiarity with much of the basic and clinical cariology research conducted over the last few decades;
- the lack of familiarity with the potential for lesions not to progress, but to stop or even regress;
- the lack of familiarity with the dynamic balance between de- and remineralization;
- financial systems for general dentists which still incentivize operative intervention over more preventive care.

These implementation challenges frequently (but not always) spread across the domains of clinical practice, dental public health and education.

References

1 Ekstrand KR, Ricketts DN, Kidd EA: Occlusal caries: pathology, diagnosis and logical management. Dent Update 2001;28:380–387.
2 Nyvad B: Diagnosis versus detection of caries. Caries Res 2004;38:192–198.
3 Zandoná AF, Zero DT: Diagnostic tools for early caries detection. J Am Dent Assoc 2006;137:1675–1684.
4 Pitts N: 'ICDAS' – an international system for caries detection and assessment being developed to facilitate caries epidemiology, research and appropriate clinical management. Community Dent Health 2004;21:193–198.
5 Ismail AI, Sohn W, Tellez M, Amaya A, Sen A, Hasson H, et al: The International Caries Detection and Assessment System (ICDAS): an integrated system for measuring dental caries. Community Dent Oral Epidemiol 2007;35:170–178.
6 Ekstrand KR, Martignon S, Ricketts DJ, Qvist V: Detection and activity assessment of primary coronal caries lesions: a methodologic study. Oper Dent 2007;32:225–235.
7 SBU: Karies – diagnostic, riskbedömning og icke-invasiv behandling. Stockholm, Swedish Council on Technology Assessment in Health Care, 2007.
8 Hume WR: Need for change in dental caries diagnosis; in Stookey GK (ed): Early Detection of Dental Caries: Proceedings of the 1st Annual Indiana Conference. Indianapolis, Indiana University School of Dentistry, 1996, pp 1–10.
9 Holmen L, Thylstrup A, Ögaard B, Kragh F: Scanning electron microscopic study of progressive stages of enamel caries in vivo. Caries Res 1985;19:355–367.
10 Holmen L, Thylstrup A, Ögaard B, Kragh F: A polarized light microscopic study of progressive stages of enamel caries in vivo. Caries Res 1985;19:348–354.
11 Holmen L, Thylstrup A, Artun J: Clinical and histological features observed during arrestment of active enamel carious lesions in vivo. Caries Res 1987;21:546–554.
12 Holmen L, Thylstrup A, Artun J: Surface changes during the arrest of active enamel carious lesions in vivo: a scanning electron microscope study. Acta Odontol Scand 1987;45:383–390.
13 Holmen L, Mejare I, Malmgren B, Thylstrup A: The effect of regular professional plaque removal on dental caries in vivo: a polarized light and scanning electron microscope study. Caries Res 1988;22:250–256.
14 Thylstrup A, Bruun C, Holmen L: In vivo caries models – mechanisms for caries initiation and arrestment. Adv Dent Res 1994;8:144–157.
15 Arends J, Christoffersen J: The nature of early caries lesions in enamel. J Dent Res 1986;65:2–11.
16 Ten Bosch JJ: Light scattering and related methods in caries diagnosis; in Stookey GK (ed): Early Detection of Dental Caries: Proceedings of the 1st Annual Indiana Conference. Indianapolis, Indiana University School of Dentistry, 1996, pp 81–90.
17 Nyvad B, Fejerskov O: Assessing the stage of caries lesion activity on the basis of clinical and microbiological examination. Community Dent Oral Epidemiol 1997;25:69–75.
18 Thylstrup A, Fejerskov O: Clinical and pathological features of dental caries; in Thylstrup A, Fejerskov O (eds): Textbook of Clinical Cariology. Copenhagen, Munksgaard, 1994, pp 111–157.
19 Bjørndal L, Thylstrup A: A structural analysis of approximal enamel caries lesions and subjacent dentin reactions. Eur J Oral Sci 1995;103:25–31.
20 Bjørndal L, Darvann T, Thylstrup A: A quantitative light microscopic study of the odontoblast and subodontoblastic reactions to active and arrested enamel caries without cavitation. Caries Res 1998;32:59–69.
21 Fejerskov O, Nyvad B: Dental caries in the aging individual; in Holm-Pedersen P, Löe H (eds): Textbook of Geriatric Dentistry. Munksgaard, Copenhagen, 1996, pp 338–372.
22 Ekstrand KR, Ricketts DNJ, Kidd EAM, Qvist V, Schou S: Detection, diagnosing, monitoring and logical treatment of occlusal caries in relation to lesion activity and severity: an in vivo examination with histological validation. Caries Res 1998;32:247–254.
23 Ekstrand KR, Bruun G, Bruun M: Plaque and gingival status as indicators for caries progression on approximal surfaces. Caries Res 1998;32:41–45.
24 Carvalho JC, Ekstrand KR, Thylstrup A: Dental plaque and caries on occlusal surfaces of first permanent molars in relation to stage of eruption. J Dent Res 1989;68:773–779.
25 Ekstrand KR, Kuzmina IN, Kuzmina E, Christiansen ME: Two and a half-year outcome of caries-preventive programs offered to groups of children in the Solntsevsky district of Moscow. Caries Res 2000;34:8–19.
26 Møller IJ: Clinical criteria for the diagnosis of the incipient carious lesion. Adv Fluor Res 1966;4:67–72.
27 Møller IJ, Poulsen S: A standardized system for diagnosing, recording and analyzing dental caries data. Scand J Dent Res 1973;81:1–11.
28 Thylstrup A, Birkeland JM: Prognosis of caries; in Thylstrup A, Fejerskov O (eds): Textbook of Cariology. Copenhagen, Munksgaard, 1986, pp 358–367.

29 Ekstrand KR, Björndal L: Structural analyses of plaque and caries in relation to the morphology of the groove-fossa system on erupting mandibular third molars. Caries Res 1997;31:336–348.

30 Carvalho JC, Ekstrand KR, Thylstrup A: Results after 1 year of non-operative occlusal caries treatment of erupting permanent first molars. Community Dent Oral Epidemiol 1991;19:23–28.

31 Fejerskov O, Thylstrup A: Different concepts of dental caries and their implications; in Thylstrup A, Fejerskov O (eds): Textbook of Clinical Cariology. Copenhagen, Munksgaard, 1994, pp 209–217.

32 Bardow A, Hofer E, Nyvad B, ten Cate JM, Kirkeby S, Moe D, Nauntofte B: Effect of saliva composition on experimental root caries. Caries Res 2005;39:71–77.

33 Carlos JP, Gittelsohn AM: Longitudinal studies of the natural history of caries II. Arch Oral Biol 1965;10:739–751.

34 Kotsanos N, Darling AI. Influence of posteruptive age of enamel on its susceptibility to artificial caries. Caries Res 1991;25:241–250.

35 Koulourides T: Implications of remineralization in the treatment of dental caries. Higashi Nippon Dental Journal 1986;5:1–20.

36 Ismail AI: Visual and visuo-tactile detection of dental caries. J Dent Res 2004;83(spec No C):C56–66.

37 Howat AP: A comparison of the sensitivity of caries diagnostic criteria. Caries Res 1981;15:331–337.

38 Pitts NB, Fyffe HE: The effect of varying diagnostic thresholds upon clinical caries data for a low prevalence group. J Dent Res 1988;67:592–596.

39 Fejerskov O, Luan WM, Nyvad B, Budtz-Jørgensen E, Holm-Pedersen P: Active and inactive root surface caries lesions in a selected group of 60- to 80-year-old Danes. Caries Res 1991;25:385–391.

40 Ismail AI, Brodeur JM, Cagnon P, Payette M, Picard D, Hamalian T, Olivier M, Eastwood BJ: Prevalence of non-cavitated and cavitated carious lesions in a random sample of 7–9-year old schoolchildren in Montreal, Quebec. Community Dent Oral Epidemiol 1992;22:250–255.

41 Rosen B, Birkedhed D, Nilsson K, Olavi O, Egelberg I: Reproducibility of clinical caries diagnoses on coronal and root surfaces. Caries Res 1996;30:1–7.

42 Amarante E, Radal M, Espelid I: Impact of diagnostic creiteria on the prevalence on dental caries in Norwegian children aged 5, 12 and 18 years. Community Dent Oral Epidemiol 1998;26:87–94.

43 Nyvad B, Machiulskiene V, Baelum V: Reliability of a new caries diagnostic system differentiating between active and inactive caries lesions. Caries Res 1999;33:252–260.

44 Fyffe HE, Deery C, Nugent ZJ, Nuttall NM, Pitts NB: In vitro validity of the Dundee Selectable Threshold Method for caries diagnosis (DSTM). Community Dent Oral Epidemiol 2000;28:52–58.

45 Nyvad B, Machiulskiene V, Baelum V: Construct and predictive validity of clinical caries diagnostic criteria assessing lesion activity. J Dent Res 2003;82:117–122.

46 Ekstrand KR, Ricketts DNJ, Longbottom C, Pitts NB: Visual and tactile assessment of arrested initial enamel carious lesions: an in vivo pilot study. Caries Res 2005;39:173–177.

47 Ekstrand KR, Martignon S, Pedersen PH: Development and evaluation of two root caries controlling programmes for home-based frail people older than 75. Gerodontology 2008;25:67–75.

48 Ekstrand KR, Ricketts DNJ, Kidd EAM: Reproducibility and accuracy of three methods for assessment of demineralization depth of the occlusal surface: an in vitro examination. Caries Res 1997;31:224–231.

49 Côrtes DF, Ekstrand KR, Elias-Boneta AR, Ellwood RP: An in vitro comparison of the ability of fibre-optic transillumination, visual inspection and radiographs to detect occlusal caries and evaluate lesion depth. Caries Res 2000;34:443–447.

50 Côrtes DF, Ellwood RP, Ekstrand KR: An in vitro comparison of a combined FOTI/visual examination of occlusal caries with other caries diagnostic methods and the effect on stain on their diagnostic performance. Caries Res 2003;37:8–16.

51 Jablonski-Momeni A, Stachniss V, Ricketts DN, Heinzel-Gutenbrunner M, Pieper K: Reproducibility and accuracy of the ICDAS-II for detection of occlusal caries in vitro. Caries Res 2008;42:79–87.

52 Hotzclaw HF, Robinson WR, Odom JD: General Chemistry, ed 9, rev. Toronto, Hearth, 1991.

53 Larsen MJ: Enamel Solubility, Caries and Erosions; thesis, Aarhus Royal Dental College, 1975.

54 Larsen MJ, Bruun C: Enamel/saliva – inorganic chemical reactions; in Thylstrup A, Fejerskov O (eds): Textbook of Cariology. Copenhagen, Munksgaard, 1986, pp 181–203.

55 Backer Dirks O: Posteruptive changes in dental enamel. J Dent Res 1966;45:503–511.

56 Maupomé G, Shulman JD, Clark DC, Levy SM, Berkowitz J: Tooth-surface progression and reversal changes in fluoridated and no-longer-fluoridated communities over a 3-year period. Caries Res 2001;35:95–110.

57 Schmid B, Fischeder D, Arndt S, Haeberlein I: Site specific detection of lactic acid production on tooth surfaces (abstract 132). Caries Res 2002;36:217.

58 Nyvad B, Fejerskov O: Active root surface caries converted into active caries as a response to oral hygiene. Scand J Dent Res 1986;94:281–284.

59 Lynch E, Beighton D: A comparison of primary root caries lesions classified according to colour. Caries Res 1994;28:233–239.
60 Özer L, Thylstrup A: What is known about caries in relation to restorations as a reason for replacement? A review. Adv Dent Res 1995;9:394–402.
61 Wulf HR: Rational Diagnosis and Treatment: An Introduction to Clinical Decision-Making, ed 2. Oxford, Blackwell Scientific Publications, 1981.
62 Wenzel A, Hintze H: The choice of gold standard for evaluating tests for caries diagnosis. Dentomaxillofac Radiol 1999;28:132–136.
63 Last JM: A Dictionary of Epidemiology, ed 4. New York, Oxford University Press, 2001.
64 Hojo S, Komatsu M, Okuda R Takahashi N, Yamada T: Acid profiles and pH of carious dentin in active and arrested lesions. J Dent Res 1994;73:1853–1857.
65 Fejerskov O: Changing paradigms in concepts on dental caries: consequences for oral health care. Caries Res 2004;38:182–191.
66 Geddes DA: Acids produced by human dental plaque metabolism in situ. Caries Res 1975;9:98–109.
67 Kingman A: Statistical issues in risk models for caries; in Bader JD (ed): Risk Assessment in Dentistry. Chapel Hill, University of North Carolina Dental Ecology, 1990, pp 193–200.

K.R. Ekstrand
University of Copenhagen
DK–2200 Copenhagen (Denmark)
Tel. +45 3532 6813, Fax +45 3532 6505, E-Mail kim@odont.ku.dk

Patient Caries Risk Assessment

Svante Twetman[a] · Margherita Fontana[b]

[a]Department of Cariology and Endodontics, Faculty of Health Sciences, University of Copenhagen, Copenhagen, Denmark; [b]Department of Preventive and Community Dentistry, Indiana University School of Dentistry, Indianapolis, Ind., USA

Abstract

Risk assessment is an essential component in the decision-making process for the correct prevention and management of dental caries. Multiple risk factors and indicators have been proposed as targets in the assessment of risk of future disease, varying sometimes based on the age group at which they are targeted. Multiple reviews and systematic reviews are available in the literature on this topic. This chapter focusses primarily on results of reviews based on longitudinal studies required to establish the accuracy of caries risk assessment. These findings demonstrate that there is a strong body of evidence to support that caries experience is still, unfortunately, the single best predictor for future caries development. In young children, prediction models which include a variety of risk factors seem to increase the accuracy of the prediction, while the usefulness of additional risk factors for prediction purposes, as measured until now in the literature, is at best questionable in schoolchildren, adolescents and adults. That is not to say these additional factors should not be assessed to help understand the strength of their associations with the disease experience in a particular patient, and aid in the development of an individualized and targeted preventive and management plan.

Copyright © 2009 S. Karger AG, Basel

Risk is defined as the probability that a harmful or unwanted event will occur, and the rationale of caries risk assessment is primarily to identify individuals with an increased risk for future disease development during a specified period of time. In addition, it would also be important to correctly identify those individuals with a risk of increased progression of the severity of the existing caries lesions. Because of the multifactorial nature of the dental caries disease process, and the fact that the disease is very dynamic but not continuous (e.g. it can progress and/or regress), studies on risk assessment tend to be complex, with a multitude of variables challenging the prediction at different times during the life of an individual (fig. 1). For a clinician the concepts of assessment of risk and prognosis are an important part of clinical decision-making. In fact, the dentist's overall subjective impression of the patient might have as good predictive power for caries risk as a detailed analysis of other factors [1].

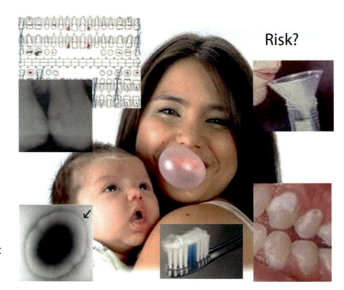

Fig. 1. Example of factors that may affect caries risk assessment.

However, a more objective assessment is desirable. The interest for such an assessment strategy was limited up to a few decades ago because the prevalence of caries was generally high in most industrialized communities. Along with the dramatic decline in caries prevalence during the past 30 years, the search for acceptable, suitable, accurate and cost-effective strategies for identifying high-risk individuals has been intensified. Furthermore, the shift from restorative therapies towards available and effective non-operative intervention strategies in prevention and early caries management has also stimulated this development.

Most reviews of the literature on this topic have concluded that 'past caries experience', and especially active existing lesions, is the most powerful single predictor of future caries development at practically all ages [2, 3]. However, from a disease management perspective this is a less than desirable outcome, considering the fact that the disease is actually manifested before it can be accurately predicted, and the ultimate goal of caries management is to prevent even the earliest enamel lesions. The aim of this chapter is to review the scientific background and grade the existing evidence for patient caries risk assessment.

Risk Factors and Risk Indicators

As caries is a multifactorial disease, a number of variables, often called risk factors, have been proposed and evaluated as tools for prediction. Usually, information on demographic, social, behavioural and biological factors from the case history, clinical/radiographic examination and supplementary tests are taken to develop a caries

Table 1. Examples of variables commonly used for an individual caries risk assessment

Variables	Quantification	High-risk values
Sociodemographic		
Socio-economic level	education level	low
Immigrant background	parent generation	mother 1st generation
Behavioural		
Mental or physical disabilities	case history	medication, impaired priority
Awareness and attitudes	interview	poor 'healthy choices'
Diet and sweet intakes	frequency	cariogenic and several times daily
Juice and soft drinks	habit and frequency	sipping and several times daily
Nocturnal meals (toddlers)	frequency	regular habit
Toothbrushing	frequency	irregular, not supervised
Fluoride exposure	frequency	non-daily
Clinical and radiographic		
Caries prevalence	dmft/DMFT	clearly higher than average for age
Proximal enamel lesions	bitewing radiographs	>2 new lesions or progressive
Oral hygiene level	visible plaque index	>50% of inspected sites
Gingival condition	bleeding on probing	>20% of measured sites
Supplementary tests		
Bacterial challenge	cultivation	high mutans streptococcus counts
Salivary secretion rate	sialometry	<0.5 ml/min (stimulated)
Salivary buffer capacity	titration	low (pH ≤4.0)

The indicated values are suggestive of a high caries risk but may vary by age and population and should be correspondingly adjusted.

risk profile or risk category [4]. Examples of background factors that may directly or indirectly influence caries risk are shown in table 1 but the list can be much longer. In fact, Harris et al. [5] identified over 100 factors associated with early childhood caries in a systematic review. Unfortunately, there is no consensus in the literature concerning the use of the terms 'risk factor' and 'risk indicator' [6, 7]. Traditionally, a risk factor plays an essential role in the aetiology of the disease, while a risk indicator is indirectly associated with the disease [8]. A risk factor can, however, be strongly associated with a disease without being useful as a predictor. For example, numerous studies have shown a positive relationship between caries and salivary mutans streptococci, but, yet, the accuracy of existing salivary tests for mutans streptococci in predicting future caries is low [9]. It is, therefore, suggested that the term 'risk factor' should be exclusively used for variables established of value for prediction purposes in prospective studies. The longitudinal design is thus required to evaluate whether or not a factor is a real risk factor, which means that it is present before the disease.

Table 2. Two-by-two table with combination of presence/absence of risk factor and disease demonstrating the calculation of sensitivity, specificity, and positive and negative predictive values

	Disease	No disease
Risk factor	a = true-positive (correct)	b = false-positive
No risk factor	c = false-negative	d = true-negative (correct)

Sensitivity = a/a + c; positive predictive value = a/a + b; specificity = d/b + d; negative predictive value = d/c + d. The values can range from 0 to 1, but are often multiplied by 100 and expressed as percent. The closer to 1, the better the risk factor. If the sum of sensitivity and specificity is 2, the risk factor is perfect. If the sensitivity and specificity are <0.5, the risk factor is not better than a guess by chance.

Consequently, the terms risk indicator/risk marker should be used for factors established in cross-sectional studies as being associated with the disease, in which correlations between various factors and the disease are investigated. A risk indicator, or combinations of several indicators, may very well be a risk factor if validated in prospective trials. Most studies dealing with caries prediction or risk assessment utilize models with several risk factors/risk indicators.

Terms Used for Caries Risk Assessment

Even if a risk assessment procedure is intended for the individual, its effectiveness must be evaluated and measured in populations. An ideal method for caries risk assessment should be inexpensive, quick and simple and have a high precision and accuracy. Most importantly, it should function as a useful aid in decision-making and determine the appropriate interval for patient recall. This means that it should be sensitive enough to catch as many as possible of those with a true caries risk but also correctly identify those with a low risk. The validation must be carried out in longitudinal studies, and the results are generally expressed in terms of sensitivity, specificity and predictive values (table 2). Sensitivity is the proportion of diseased subjects with a positive risk factor while specificity denotes the proportion of non-diseased subjects whose risk factor is negative. The predictive values are perhaps of greater interest for the clinician since they express the probability of an individual with a positive or negative risk factor to develop or avoid future disease. The combined value of sensitivity and specificity describes the precision or reliability of a risk factor, and a sum of at least 1.6% has been proposed as the least acceptable level for clinically relevant prediction models [10]. This level has, however, been almost impossible to achieve in schoolchildren and elderly individuals, even in the most ambitious attempts with over 20 risk variables [1]. Furthermore, it is important to keep in mind that while the values of sensitivity and specificity are quite stable, the predictive values cannot be generalized from one population to another.

They are highly dependent on factors such as the prevalence and incidence of caries, criteria for collecting data, cut-off values, and the number and or combination of risk factors or tests applied. For example, with a lower caries prevalence in a population, the positive predictive value decreases at a given sensitivity and specificity.

In the scientific literature there is a range of other measures used to describe the accuracy of caries risk assessment. Some studies report the relative risk and the odds ratio values, referring to the chance of an event (e.g. caries) versus a non-event (e.g. no caries). Others use the likelihood ratio, which is a measure that summarizes the sensitivity and specificity independently of the prevalence of the disease. Receiver-operating characteristic with area under the curve is a common way to graphically illustrate the outcome of a risk assessment.

Evidence for Caries Risk Assessment

As already discussed, longitudinal studies are required to establish the accuracy of caries risk assessment. Unfortunately, there are few such studies of good quality available, especially in adults, and previous systematic reviews have, therefore, been forced to mostly rely on correlation studies [5, 9, 11]. In 2007, a task group within the Swedish Council on Technology Assessment in Health Care presented a systematic review of caries risk assessment procedures at different ages [12] (www.sbu.se) based on prospective longitudinal trials. Retrospective studies were included only in the event they were of high quality with low risk for bias or confounders. Among the main inclusion criteria, an adequately described and selected study group exceeding 70 patients was demanded, and a 2-year follow-up was required for permanent teeth while 1 year was sufficient for the primary dentition. Moreover, the risk factors as well as the caries diagnostic criteria had to be clearly defined, with reported endpoints of sensitivity and specificity, relative risk, odds ratio or receiver-operating characteristic. The search strategies in Medline and Pubmed identified over 800 original papers, and approximately 200 were examined in full text. In addition, 5 systematic reviews and 22 narrative reviews were identified during the search. After strictly applying the inclusion criteria, 63 papers were independently assessed by 2 reviewers, and the quality was graded as high, medium or low according to the predetermined criteria. Due to the heterogeneity of the risk factors used, the main findings are reported below according to age or risk factor. A grading of recommendations for clinical use according to the Scottish Dental Clinical Effectiveness Programme is shown in table 3.

Findings for Toddlers and Preschool Children

Out of the 19 studies that met the inclusion criteria, 5 studies, published in 7 papers, were graded as being of medium or high quality [13–19]. Collectively the papers showed

Table 3. Risk factors for caries risk assessment – grading of recommendations according to the Scottish Dental Clinical Effectiveness Programme

Risk factor	Age group	Recommendation
Past/current caries experience	all ages	R_s
Prediction models including several factors	preschool children	R_s
Sugar intake	all ages	R_w
Enumeration of caries-associated bacteria	all ages	R_w
Visible plaque	toddlers	R_w
Fluoride exposure	preschool children	R_w
Posteruptive age	young permanent dentition	R_s
Saliva flow rate, buffer capacity	all ages	R_e

R_s = Recommendations supported by strong evidence with limited bias; R_w = recommendations supported by weak evidence with some potential for bias; R_e = recommendations based on expert opinion.

that the possibilities to correctly identify preschool children at risk are relatively high, and they displayed strong evidence that the predictive ability increased if models with a combination of several risk factors were used. For example, at 1 year of age, a combination of sociodemographic factors, dietary habits and mutans streptococcus counts gave a sensitivity and specificity sum of 1.7% [14]. A follow-up analysis when the same children were 2.5 years of age showed, however, that the presence of caries lesions was now the single best predictor [15]. Notably, the study was performed in a low socio-economic immigrant area in Sweden with a relatively high prevalence of caries. In another study of toddlers from Finland [19], the greatest precision in prediction was achieved by a combination of history of caries lesions, dietary habits and mutans streptococci, with the latter being the best single predictor (sensitivity 0.69, specificity 0.78). Both Nordic studies found a significant correlation between caries lesion development and frequent consumption of products containing sugar, but the predictive power of this variable was limited with a high sensitivity but a poor specificity.

The presence of mutans streptococci or lactobacilli in saliva or plaque as a sole predictor for caries in the primary dentition was also evaluated in the above-mentioned studies. However, the accuracy of these measurements was shown to be low, with either a low sensitivity combined with high specificity or vice versa. Likewise, the presence of visual plaque on the labial surfaces of the front teeth of toddlers was tested as a predictor for the development of caries lesions during the following 2–3 years, but again with poor accuracy. Wendt et al. [16] followed children from 1 to 3 years of age and showed that those who brushed their teeth daily with fluoride toothpaste had a 3 times higher chance to remain 'caries free' at the age of 3 compared with those with poor oral hygiene. Three studies investigated the ability to predict caries lesions based on the presence of caries in the primary dentition either alone or in combination with other risk factors [20–22]. The studies were heterogeneous and displayed different predictive potentials. Nevertheless, the average values were 0.62 for sensitivity and 0.79 for specificity.

Findings for Schoolchildren and Adolescents

Thirty studies were initially included, but only 5 were appraised as high or medium quality [1, 23–26]. Despite the limited comparability between the studies, it was obvious that the current caries status, as a result of past caries activity, was the most effective predictive factor. However, in contrast to the youngest children, there was strong evidence that the chance to correctly identify non-risk individuals was greater than a correct identification of individuals with high risk. The calculated mean value of sensitivity was 0.61, and the corresponding value of specificity was 0.82. The use of additional risk factors such as plaque, bacterial tests, salivary factors and exposure to fluoride did not markedly improve the predictive power. This may be explained in part by the fact that the current level of caries experience reflects relatively well both past and current interplay between the various aetiological factors. In the studies, as well as in a systematic review [27], it was noted that the association between sugar intake and caries lesions today was much less marked than it used to be. Consequently, in schoolchildren and teenagers from low-caries-risk populations with a daily use of fluoride toothpaste, daily consumption of sugary snacks between meals is not particularly useful in caries prediction models. However, because of the integral role that sugars play in the development of dental caries, a dietary analysis still remains an important element in the development of an individualized patient-centred caries management protocol.

Findings for Posteruptive Age as a Predictor

Six longitudinal studies were initially included in the search, of which 3 were rated to be of high or medium quality [28–30]. Those studies revealed strong scientific evidence that the risk of developing caries in permanent teeth is greatest during the years immediately after eruption. For occlusal surfaces, the first molars are at greatest risk during the first year, and the second molars during the first 2–3 years after eruption. The approximal surfaces are at greatest risk during the first 3–4 years after eruption.

Findings for Prediction of Root Caries in Adults

Thirteen papers were included for this topic, of which 3, focusing on root caries, were of medium quality [31–33]. Collectively, the studies presented limited evidence that previous experience of root caries, loss of periodontal attachment and presence of salivary lactobacilli may increase the risk for future root caries. The accuracy with these risk factors exhibited great variability in the different trials. No prospective studies were identified with the aim to predict coronal caries development in adults, or to assess the impact of hyposalivation/dry mouth on caries risk. It is, however, well known that a normal salivary function is essential for dental health and that a low salivary flow rate is associated with increased caries risk [34]. Therefore, managing salivary flow rate is important in the management of dental caries, but there is lack of evidence from longitudinal studies to suggest at this point that this is a strong stand-alone predictor of future caries experience in adults.

Conclusions and Comments

Caries risk assessment is one of the cornerstones in patient-centred caries management. An assessment of the patient's risk factors and indicators should help both the prediction of future caries (in this case only proven predictive factors should be considered) and the identification of factors that affect caries development. This, in turn, should influence a tailored caries management plan by affecting the decision-making process regarding type of treatment(s) needed (i.e. surgical and/or non-surgical), intensity/frequency of treatment(s), frequency of recall appointments, and need for additional diagnostic procedures [35]. Based on longitudinal studies, there is a strong body of evidence that past caries experience (or present caries activity) is the single best predictor for future caries development, with additional factors increasing the accuracy, in some instances, only when applied to very young children. It is important to note, however, that weak evidence, or even lack of evidence from clinical trials, does not necessarily mean that the variety of risk factors and indicators that are available for the clinician's consideration should be abandoned. As previously pointed out, the reason for non-existing evidence is most often lack of studies of good quality. For example, plaque amount and tooth morphology may very well be risk factors, although not yet established in an adequate prospective way. Furthermore, as mentioned earlier, the 'gut feeling' among dental professionals, which is impossible to define, is a factor that should not be underestimated as shown in the North Carolina risk study [1]. Therefore, we argue that at this point it is more important that a risk assessment is carried out, incorporating the best available evidence, than that no attempt is made due to the lack of firm evidence. The risk should be documented in a patient's chart and used to influence a treatment plan. As a didactic aid for patient motivation, an interactive computer-based risk assessment program can be used in order to illustrate the relative importance of various background factors in an individual risk profile [36] as shown in figure 2.

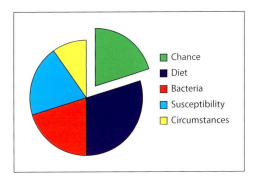

Fig. 2. Cariogram – a validated interactive program for patient motivation [36]. Factors of importance for the caries process are entered and weighted, together forming a caries risk profile for the patient. The sector set apart is the 'chance of avoiding caries in the near future', expressed as percent. The program can be downloaded at www.db.mah.se/car/cariogram.

Future Considerations

An important outcome of systematic reviews is to identify areas of future research. Obviously, new risk factors could be identified, but it is more likely and feasible to suggest that methods for evaluating existing risk factors and indicators will be further developed as new molecular and genetic chair side strategies become possible. However, probably the most urgent need in clinical practice today is a validated way to objectively assess caries activity. Of great importance is also the realization that the majority of the body of evidence in caries risk assessment comes from studies on primary or permanent teeth in children and adolescents, with very few studies in the elderly and almost no studies in young adults. Furthermore, to allow the body of evidence to grow, and provide for strong conclusions and recommendations in the future, it is important to suggest that future studies are carefully reviewed in order to achieve a better homogenous design with comparable predictors, cut-off points and statistical analysis as well as outcome measures. Finally, studies that assess whether use of a risk-based caries management plan is cost-effective and results in improved health are a challenge for the future.

Acknowledgements

The authors would like to acknowledge the SBU project group behind the systematic review on caries risk assessment [12] on which parts of this paper are based: Dr. Ingegerd Mejàre (head), Dr. Susanna Axelsson, Dr. Gunnar Dahlén, Dr. Ivar Espelid, Dr. Anders Norlund, Dr. Sofia Tranæus and Dr. Svante Twetman.

References

1 Disney JA, Graves RC, Stamm JW, Bohannan HM, Abernathy JR, Zack DD: The University of North Carolina Caries Risk Assessment Study: further developments in caries risk prediction. Community Dent Oral Epidemiol 1992;20:64–75.

2 Demers M, Brodeur JM, Simard PL, Mouton C, Veilleux G, Fréchette S: Caries predictors suitable for mass-screenings in children: a literature review. Community Dent Health 1990;7:11–21.

3 Powell LV: Caries prediction: a review of the literature. Community Dent Oral Epidemiol 1998;26:361–371.
4 Burt BA: Definitions of risk. J Dent Educ 2001;65:1007–1008.
5 Harris R, Nicoll AD, Adair PM, Pine CM: Risk factors for dental caries in young children: a systematic review of the literature. Community Dent Health 2004;21:71–85.
6 Beck JD: Risk revisited. Community Dent Oral Epidemiol 1998;26:220–225.
7 Burt BA: Concepts of risk in dental public health. Community Dent Oral Epidemiol 2005;33:240–247.
8 Rothman KJ: Modern Epidemiology. Boston, Little, Brown & Co, 1986.
9 Thenisch NL, Bachmann IM, Imfeld T, Leisebach Minder T, Steurer J: Are mutans streptococci detected in preschool children a reliable predictive factor for dental caries risk? A systematic review. Caries Res 2006;40:366–374.
10 Kingman A: Statistical in risk models for caries; in Bader J (ed): Risk Assessment in Dentistry. Chapel Hill, University of North Carolina Dental Ecology, 1990, pp 193–200.
11 Zero D, Fontana M, Lennon AM: Clinical applications and outcomes of using indicators of risk in caries management. J Dent Educ 2001;65:1132–1138.
12 SBU: Caries – diagnosis, risk assessment and non-invasive treatment. A systematic review. Summary and conclusions. Report No 188. Stockholm, Swedish Council on Technology Assessment in Health Care, 2007.
13 Demers M, Brodeur JM, Mouton C, Simard PL, Trahan L, Veilleux G: A multivariate model to predict caries increment in Montreal children aged 5 years. Community Dent Health 1992;9:273–281.
14 Grindefjord M, Dahllöf G, Nilsson B, Modéer T: Prediction of dental caries development in 1-year-old children. Caries Res 1995;29:343–348.
15 Grindefjord M, Dahllöf G, Nilsson B, Modéer T: Stepwise prediction of dental caries in children up to 3.5 years of age. Caries Res 1996;30:256–266.
16 Wendt LK, Hallonsten AL, Koch G, Birkhed D: Analysis of caries-related factors in infants and toddlers living in Sweden. Acta Odontol Scand 1996;54:131–137.
17 Karjalainen S, Söderling E, Sewón L, Lapinleimu H, Simell O: A prospective study on sucrose consumption, visible plaque and caries in children from 3 to 6 years of age. Community Dent Oral Epidemiol 2001;29:136–142.
18 Pienihäkkinen K, Jokela J: Clinical outcomes of risk-based caries prevention in preschool-aged children. Community Dent Oral Epidemiol 2002;30:143–150.
19 Pienihäkkinen K, Jokela J, Alanen P: Assessment of caries risk in preschool children. Caries Res 2004;38:156–162.
20 Stewart PW, Stamm JW: Classification tree prediction models for dental caries from clinical, microbiological, and interview data. J Dent Res 1991;70:1239–1251.
21 Vanobbergen J, Martens L, Lesaffre E, Bogaerts K, Declerck D: The value of a baseline caries risk assessment model in the primary dentition for the prediction of caries incidence in the permanent dentition. Caries Res 2001;35:442–450.
22 Skeie MS, Raadal M, Strand GV, Espelid I: The relationship between caries in the primary dentition at 5 years of age and permanent dentition at 10 years of age – a longitudinal study. Int J Paediatr Dent 2006;16:152–160.
23 Russel JI, MacFarlane TW, Aitchison TC, Stephen KW, Burchell CK: Prediction of caries increment in Scottish adolescents. Community Dent Oral Epidemiol 1991;19:74–77.
24 Burt BA, Szpunar SM: The Michigan Study: the relationship between sugars intake and dental caries over three years. Int Dent J 1994;44:230–240.
25 Vanobbergen J, Martens L, Lesaffre E, Bogaerts K, Declerck D: Assessing risk indicators for dental caries in the primary dentition. Community Dent Oral Epidemiol 2001;29:424–439.
26 Stenlund H, Mejáre I, Källestål C: Caries rates related to approximal caries at ages 11–13: a 10-year follow-up study. J Dent Res 2002;81:455–458.
27 Burt BA, Pai S: Sugar consumption and caries risk: a systematic review. J Dent Educ 2001;65:1017–1023.
28 Abernathy JR, Graves RC, Greenberg BG, Bohannan HM, Disney JA: Application of life table methodology in determining dental caries rates. Community Dent Oral Epidemiol 1986;14:261–264.
29 Baelum V, Machiulskiene V, Nyvad B, Richards A, Vaeth M: Application of survival analysis to caries lesion transitions in intervention trials. Community Dent Oral Epidemiol 2003;31:252–230.
30 Mejáre I, Stenlund H, Zelezny-Holmlund C: Caries incidence and lesion progression from adolescence to young adulthood: a prospective 15-year cohort study in Sweden. Caries Res 2004;38:130–131.
31 Beck JD, Kohout F, Hunt RJ: Identification of high caries risk adults: attitudes, social factors and diseases. Int Dent J 1988;38:231–238.
32 Gilbert GH, Duncan RP, Dolan TA, Forester U: Twenty-four month incidence of root caries among a diverse group of adults. Caries Res 2001;35:366–375.

33 Takano N, Ando Y, Yoshihara A, Miyazaki H: Factors associated with root caries incidence in an elderly population. Community Dent Health 2003; 20:217–222.
34 Leone CW, Oppenheim FG: Physical and chemical aspects of saliva as indicators of risk for dental caries in humans. J Dent Educ 2001;65:1054–1062.
35 Fontana M, Zero DT: Assessing patient's caries risk. J Am Dent Assoc 2006;137:1231–1239.
36 Hänsel Petersson G, Twetman S, Bratthall D: Evaluation of a computer program for caries risk assessment in schoolchildren. Caries Res 2002;36: 327–340.

S. Twetman
Department of Cariology and Endodontics, Faculty of Health Sciences, University of Copenhagen
Nørre Allé 20
DK–2200 Copenhagen N (Denmark)
Tel. +45 3532 6810, Fax +45 3532 6700, E-Mail stw@odont.ku.dk

Dentition and Lesion History

H. Eggertsson · A. Ferreira-Zandona

Indiana University School of Dentistry, Indianapolis, Ind., USA

Abstract

Dental caries is a process that typically keeps recurring throughout life, and the consequences are too often seen as irreversible damage to the dentition. At various stages of life, different parts of the dentition are affected, and the effects continue to be seen in the dentition long after the events took place. They bear witness to previous occurrences of this process throughout the lifetime of an individual. This chapter reviews the linkage between the caries process and the dental caries lesion history of the human dentition. The prevalence and distribution of the caries burden are very variable and closely tied to cultural aspects. In the primary dentition, income and education have been found to be inversely associated with: (1) any early childhood caries and (2) the maxillary incisor caries pattern. A positive association between these caries patterns and minority ethnicity/race status was also identified. These patterns are different from those of the permanent dentition. Well-documented changes in caries prevalence have been observed throughout history, most closely tied to availability and amount of refined sugar consumed. Changes in caries rates are also well documented in the 20th century, mainly with the advent of fluoride in several forms, first as a steep decline and recently as being relatively unchanged. It is likely that there will be dramatic changes in the rates and distribution of dental caries in the future, due to changes in behavioural factors and therapeutic measures. The description drawn is based on the dental caries pattern experienced in modern western societies.

Copyright © 2009 S. Karger AG, Basel

Dental caries is a process that keeps recurring throughout life, and the consequences are too often seen as irreversible damage to the dentition. At various stages of life, different parts of the dentition are being affected, and the effects continue to be seen in the dentition long after the events took place. They bear witness to previous occurrences of this process throughout the lifetime of an individual. This chapter will review the linkage of the caries process and the dental caries lesion history of the human dentition.

The prevalence and distribution of the caries burden are very variable and closely tied to cultural aspects [1, 2]. In the primary dentition, income and education have been found to be inversely associated with: (1) any early childhood caries (ECC) and (2) the maxillary incisor caries pattern. A positive association between these caries patterns and minority ethnicity/race status was also identified [3]. These patterns are different from those of the permanent dentition [4]. Three additional caries intra-oral patterns demonstrated more varied associations with socio-economic status, ethnicity/race and income and education [3, 5].

Although caries as a process can be traced back to early hominids [6], at various times in the history of the human race caries has been an almost unknown disease [7, 8]. Well-documented changes in caries prevalence have been observed throughout history, most closely tied to availability and amount consumed of refined sugar [9]. Changes in caries rates are also well documented in the 20th century, mainly with the advent of fluoride in several forms, first as a steep decline and recently as being relatively unchanged [10]. It is likely that there will be dramatic changes in the rates and distribution of dental caries in the future due to changes in behavioural factors and therapeutic measures. The following description is based on the dental caries pattern experienced in modern western societies, as most of the available information comes from there. This discussion will be divided into the primary dentition and the permanent dentition. Although there are several similarities between the dentitions, there are also some important differences.

Establishing the Oral Flora

Much focus has been placed on mutans streptococci as a main pathogenic agent in dental caries. Theoretically, streptococcal colonization can begin as soon as a few square millimeters of the incisal edges of primary teeth become visible. It has been postulated that the earlier the establishment of mutans streptococci in the plaque of the primary teeth, the earlier and more extensive the caries development [11].

The acquisition of mutans streptococci in young children has been suggested to take place during a 'window of infectivity', with the age range reported varying between 3 and 31 months of age. Studies have linked, with different levels of confidence, the acquisition of mutans streptococci and the prevalence of dental caries [12, 13]. *Streptococcus mutans* colonization has been found in predentate infants as young as 3 months of age with prevalences ranging from 20 to 34% [12, 13]. *S. mutans* has also been found to be positively associated with numbers of developmental nodules in a dose-response relationship ($p < 0.001$), and with maternal salivary levels of the bacteria ($p = 0.03$) [12].

Based on the 'window of infectivity' hypothesis, attempts have been made to reduce levels of salivary mutans streptococci in pregnant women with the aim of subsequently inhibiting the growth of these bacteria in their young children [14, 15]. In a 30-month study [14], beginning at the end of the sixth month of pregnancy and continuing until delivery, subjects rinsed their mouths daily with 0.05% sodium fluoride and 0.12% chlorhexidine. This treatment significantly reduced salivary mutans streptococcus levels in mothers and delayed the colonization of bacteria in their children for about 4 months. Turksel Dulgergil et al. [15] similarly demonstrated, in a 24-month study, that a preventive regimen in mothers in a test group led to a significant reduction in mutans streptococci and lactobacilli in plaque ($p < 0.001$), whereas no such trend was observed in control children during the 24-month monitoring period ($p > 0.05$). Turksel Dulgergil et al. also examined the occurrence of caries (dfs) after 12 months and found it to be significantly lower in the test group than in the control group (0.13 ± 0.35 vs. 1.67 ± 1.30, respectively; $p < 0.001$). A similar difference was observed after 24 months (0.2 ± 0.56 vs. 3.17 ± 1.70, respectively; $p < 0.001$).

Another approach to prevent colonization has been focused on immune responses. The initial infection of children by *S. mutans* depends on its ability to adhere and accumulate on tooth surfaces. These processes involve the adhesin antigen I/II, glucosyltransferases and glucan-binding protein B, each a target for anticaries vaccines. Salivary immunoglobulin A antibody responses to *S. mutans* antigens have been detected from 6 months of age indicating that immunoglobulin A antibody specificities may be critical in modulating initial *S. mutans* infection [16].

Pattern of Caries in the Primary Dentition

The pattern of caries is different in the primary and permanent dentition [4].

ECC is defined as the presence of one or more decayed (non-cavitated/cavitated lesions), missing or filled tooth surfaces in a child under 6 years of age (American Academy of Pediatric Dentistry, 2008) while any sign of smooth-surface caries in a child younger than 36 months of age indicates severe ECC. Four caries patterns have been suggested for the primary dentition: (i) any maxillary incisor surfaces, (ii) first molar occlusal surfaces, (iii) second molar pit-and-fissure surfaces and (iv) any smooth surfaces, excluding the maxillary incisor surfaces [17–19].

At the population level there is indication that caries experience might be symmetrical in the deciduous dentition, appearing to be strongest for the left-right pairs in the mandible, followed by the left-right pairs in the maxilla. At the individual level, lesions tend to cluster on one side of the mouth [20]. Prevalence is higher in the mandibular arch and in posterior teeth followed by maxillary anterior teeth, second molars showing the higher caries prevalence [21, 22]. Wyne et al. [23] indicated that in severe ECC the teeth most affected by caries are usually maxillary central incisors, whereas the least affected are mandibular canines. There is also a high probability of bilateral molar caries [24] especially in mandibular first molars [23]. In the primary dentition, caries on occlusal and on smooth surfaces accounted each for 40% of the caries experience [25].

Absence of interdental space has been found to be only weakly associated with greater caries experience in the primary dentition [26].

Pattern of Caries in the Permanent Dentition

Different morphological tooth types are at different risk for developing caries lesions, with molars being most susceptible and lower incisors being the least susceptible. The great reduction in caries prevalence in the latter part of the last century has had a remarkably little effect on the relative susceptibility of different tooth types. In a 1941 study, Klein and Palmer identified 5 classes of susceptibility, with the mandibular molars being most attacked, followed by maxillary molars, then mandibular second premolars along with maxillary incisors and premolars, then mandibular first premolars and maxillary canines, and finally mandibular incisors and canines. Using data from the National Health and Nutrition Examination Survey III (1988–1994), Macek et al. [27] replicated in 2003 the Klein and Palmer analysis (but not their sampling method or caries scoring criteria) and found a remarkably similar pattern. They divided the susceptibility into 6 classes, with mandibular second molars being the most susceptible, followed by maxillary molars and mandibular first molar, then maxillary and mandibular second premolars, then maxillary and mandibular first premolars, then maxillary incisors, and finally mandibular incisors along with maxillary and mandibular canines. The former study took place while caries rates were high and before the implementation of preventive measures such as fluoride and sealants. The use of sealants may explain why second molars were found to be most susceptible in the second study, as the first molars are more likely to receive sealants [28]. Radiographic studies indicate a similar pattern of susceptibility with the first molar usually found to carry the majority of the caries burden, or up to 60% of total DFS [29].

Eruption Stages and Pattern of Caries in the Primary Dentition

The pattern of dental caries development is related to age and eruption and exfoliation patterns. It has been shown by cross-sectional studies and longitudinal studies that in malnourished children the pattern of caries development as a function of age is significantly altered as a result of a delayed eruption and exfoliation of the deciduous teeth [30, 31], and even mild to moderate malnutrition episode occurring during the first year of life is associated with increased caries in both the deciduous and permanent teeth many years later [31].

Impact of Primary Dentition Caries Experience

Caries experience in the primary dentition has been found to be significantly correlated with caries experience in the permanent dentition [32], specifically caries experience in primary second molar and permanent teeth [33]. It is also correlated with future caries development in the primary dentition, children presenting with posterior approximal caries and buccal lingual caries having 3 and 4 times greater dmfs in 2 years than apparently 'caries-free' children, increments also being 8 times greater [34].

Permanent Molars and Eruption Time

At the time of emergence of the posterior teeth the fissures are filled with cell remnants and connective tissue protein. These are quickly supplemented with salivary protein in the form of acquired pellicle, then other molecules and bacteria, and finally with a fully developed biofilm [35, 36]. Posteruptive changes in enamel include an increase in mineral content, in organic ions and in fluoride, all of which act to make the enamel stronger and more resistant to acid dissolution.

The eruption time of the permanent molars has been described as a particularly vulnerable period due to physical limitations on oral hygiene practices and lack of maturation of the enamel [37]. Many of the occlusal surfaces of erupting molars show signs of early lesion formation, which later revert to an arrested state or fall below the level of detection again [38]. The time for eruption plays an important role, as it is estimated that it takes the first molars on average 15 months from breaking through the oral mucosa until they have reached functional occlusion, and 27 months for the second molars, however with a large variation in eruption time for either first or second molars [39]. Relatively scarce data are available on the caries susceptibility of the third molars, but due to their posterior position and morphologically rich presentation they have been considered caries prone. The available data point however to a susceptibility similar to those of the first and second molars [40, 41].

Caries Susceptibility of Tooth Surfaces

Of all the surfaces in the mouth, the occlusal surfaces of the molars are the most susceptible [42–50]. The pattern holds true for studies predating the widespread use of fluoride and more recent ones. In recent years, the proportion of occlusal caries has increased relative to the approximal and smooth-surface caries. The occlusal molar surfaces remain the most common sites of caries attack during childhood and adolescence [46] and even into adulthood [44], and they are the surfaces least affected by the benefits of fluoride [42]. In other studies, those teeth are often quickly sealed, thereby skewing the results. A few years posteruptively, the finding of approximal lesions becomes more common [48]. There is some indication that the caries incidence slows down in some populations once young adulthood is reached [51]. Radiographic studies indicate the most susceptible tooth surface for the adolescent age group being the distal aspect of the first molars [52].

Root surfaces only become vulnerable to caries attack in adult years, and the risk increases with age. Conditions often accompanying aging contribute to the increase in prevalence of root caries, such as recession of gingival tissue, decreased salivary flow (a common side effect of multiple medications) and changes in the composition of the saliva. Although root caries is most commonly thought of on buccal surfaces, appproximal root surface lesions can present formidable restorative challenges.

Cavitated versus Non-Cavitated Lesions

Most historical data were collected using traditional caries scoring systems, which scored only lesion presence or absence at the level of cavitation. In many countries it is only in recent years that data have been collected on non-cavitated lesions. The emerging picture is that for every cavitated or filled surface in the mouth there seem to be 2 non-cavitated lesions [53, Agustsdottir, pers. commun.]. Without knowledge of the activity of those lesions, it is hard to estimate the significance of those findings. A frequent clinical finding is a narrow band of arrested white- or brown-spot lesions which are no longer in a plaque stagnation area. Those lesions are nothing but old scars, indicating that at one time the caries risk of that surface or individual was greater than under current conditions.

Speed of Progression

Earlier studies noted that there were few carious lesions detected in the first year after eruption but a burst of activity was noted 2–3 years thereafter [49]. This may be due to detection methods recording only at the level of cavitation because, when non-cavitated lesions are recorded, lesions are detected even shortly after eruption [37]. Previous studies using visual or visual-tactile methods have been incapable of monitoring lesion progression, but radiographic studies have been used to track the speed that it takes lesions to penetrate through the dental tissues. The progression speed is different within enamel from that once the lesion reaches dentine. The mean annual caries rate for formation of new lesions in a low-risk group of 11- to 22-year-olds was 3.9/100 surfaces, from the inner half of enamel into dentine 5.4/100, and, once a lesion had reached the dentine, annual progression was found in 20.3/100 surfaces [54]. The rate shows great variation according to caries risk [55] and the presence of a lesion on an adjacent approximal surface [52]. As the individuals become older, the caries rate typically, but not invariably, slows down, as indicated by slower mean progression with increasing posteruptive age [56] and with slower mean progression in adults [57].

Progression of lesions in the primary dentition has been associated with fluoride exposure, socio-economic status and beverage consumption [58]. Progression of non-cavitated lesions is more prevalent in pit-and-fissure lesions than in smooth-surface lesions [58].

Effect of the Dental Arches and Malocclusion and Enamel Hypoplasia

Not only are the molar teeth the most morphologically complex teeth, but also the ones furthest into the mouth and therefore the hardest to reach during oral hygiene procedures. The curves of the dentition also make it harder for individuals to reach the most posterior teeth or some areas of them, notably the lingual side of the lower molars, and due to the mandibular ramus, the buccal side of the upper second molars. Those areas become prone to plaque accumulation and possible lesion formation; especially the upper second molars being in a position more superior and median than their corresponding first molars, those teeth become extremely hard to maintain in a clean state, and lesions are frequent on occlusal and buccal surfaces even shortly after eruption. The lesions on the buccal surfaces of the upper second molars are different from other smooth-surface lesions in that they do not always form at the gingival margin but sometimes in the middle of the buccal surface.

Crowding of teeth, displacement and other causes of badly aligned teeth have been said to lead to increased plaque retention and greater caries experience although there is limited evidence to support this. Malocclusion may also lead to such conditions and also to conditions of mouth breathing which is associated with increased caries. Teeth in malocclusion can in some cases lead to lesions forming in unusual locations, sometimes with drastic results [59].

Hypoplasia and a highly cariogenic diet [60] have been found to be significant independent predictors of white-spot lesions or enamel cavitations, with odds 9.6 times greater for children with any hypoplasia and 7.8 times greater for children with highly cariogenic diets relative to those with lower scores, after adjusting for the level of *S. mutans,* age and ethnicity [13].

Lesion History

In the development of caries lesions, the lesions undergo cycles of demineralization and remineralization. Only when the net effect of these cycles over a given time span is demineralization is a lesion formed. However, the process may also reverse, mainly while the surface of the lesion is still intact.

Lesion Arrest or Remineralization?

While there is debate going on in some circles as to the extent to which lesions can actually remineralize in vivo, the argument is that they most certainly can remineralize under laboratory conditions, even dentine lesions can be remineralized in that way [61]. However, when all the organic material in the mouth is considered, much of which has the potential for preventing further crystal growth, the hurdles for clinical remineralization are greater. Therefore, the process named remineralization of lesions may often be more correctly named lesion arrest. Most of the mineralization during the process takes place in the surface layer, which effectively becomes blocked to further diffusion of ions in and out of the body of the lesion. Therefore it is questionable whether such a complete mineralization can occur under in vivo conditions. However, longitudinal radiographic data, assessed objectively from serial standardized radiographs, has shown lesion regression and increases in radiopacity in vivo [62].

The concept of remineralization in the clinical situation is mainly built on the classical work of Backer Dirks [63] from 1966, where the fates of white-spot lesions detected in a population participating in a water fluoridation study, with the subjects examined clinically at the age of 8 and again at the age of 15, are described. A number of the white-spot lesions noted at the age of 8 had disappeared during the second examination. It was stated that this could be due to abrasion of the lesions instead of remineralization [64] although the lesions observed by these workers had been induced by an unusually aggressive cariogenic challenge and may have been atypically softened.

Other studies indicate that lesions formed around orthodontic brackets do regress in size when measured quantitatively with quantitative light-induced fluorescence [65]. The regression may be due to abrasion, but as optical methods were used in this study, it is tempting to explore further what happens during lesion arrest. With increased deposition of minerals in the lesion area and reduction in pore size of the arrested lesion, the refractive index of the lesion area decreases, the lesion becomes more translucent and light is less scattered.

Such changes are also observed during clinical examination of the arrested lesion and form part of the basis for lesion activity assessment, where the surface is judged to be shiny in appearance. Other changes in the arrested lesion refer to the abrasion, regarding the smoothness of the lesion measured with a tactile sense using the side of an explorer [66]. There is some indication from in vitro studies that an arrested lesion is going to be more acid resistant to future acid attack than virgin enamel [67].

References

1 Shigli K, Hebbal M, Angadi GS: Relative contribution of caries and periodontal disease in adult tooth loss among patients reporting to the institute of dental sciences, Belgaum, India. Gerodontology 2008, E-pub ahead of print.
2 Rose EK, Vieira AR: Caries and periodontal disease: insights from two US populations living a century apart. Oral Health Prev Dent 2008;6:23–28.
3 Psoter WJ, Pendrys DG, Morse DE, Zhang H, Mayne ST: Associations of ethnicity/race and socioeconomic status with early childhood caries patterns. J Public Health Dent 2006;66:23–29.
4 Kaste LM, Selwitz RH, Oldakowski RJ, Brunelle JA, Winn DM, Brown LJ: Coronal caries in the primary and permanent dentition of children and adolescents 1–17 years of age: United States, 1988–1991. J Dent Res 1996;75(spec iss):631–641.

5 Angelillo IF, Anfosso R, Nobile CG, Pavia M: Prevalence of dental caries in schoolchildren in Italy. Eur J Epidemiol 1998;14:351–357 (erratum published in Eur J Epidemiol 1998;14:733).

6 Grine FE, Gwinnett AJ, Oaks JH: Early hominid dental pathology: interproximal caries in 1.5 million-year-old *Paranthropus robustus* from Swartkrans. Arch Oral Biol 1990;35:381–386.

7 Polo-Cerda M, Romero A, Casabo J, De Juan J: The bronze age burials from Cova dels Blaus (Vall d'Uixo, Castello, Spain): an approach to palaeodietary reconstruction through dental pathology, occlusal wear and buccal microwear patterns. Homo 2007;58:297–307.

8 Caglar E, Kuscu OO, Sandalli N, Ari I: Prevalence of dental caries and tooth wear in a Byzantine population (13th c. AD) from northwest Turkey. Arch Oral Biol 2007;52:1136–1145.

9 Gustafsson BE, Quensel CE, Lanke LS, Lundqvist C, Grahnen H, Bonow BE, Krasse B: The Vipeholm Dental Caries Study: the effect of different levels of carbohydrate intake on caries activity in 436 individuals observed for five years. Acta Odontol Scand 1954;11:232–264.

10 Stecksen-Blicks C, Sunnegardh K, Borssen E: Caries experience and background factors in 4-year-old children: time trends 1967–2002. Caries Res 2004;38:149–155.

11 Suhonen J: Mutans streptococci and their specific oral target: new implications to prevent dental caries? Schweiz Monatsschr Zahnmed 1992;102:286–291.

12 Wan AK, Seow WK, Walsh LJ, Bird P, Tudehope DL, Purdie DM: Association of *Streptococcus mutans* infection and oral developmental nodules in predentate infants. J Dent Res 2001;80:1945–1948.

13 Milgrom P, Riedy CA, Weinstein P, Tanner AC, Manibusan L, Bruss J: Dental caries and its relationship to bacterial infection, hypoplasia, diet, and oral hygiene in 6- to 36-month-old children. Community Dent Oral Epidemiol 2000;28:295–306.

14 Brambilla E, Felloni A, Gagliani M, Malerba A, Garcia-Godoy F, Strohmenger L: Caries prevention during pregnancy: results of a 30-month study. J Am Dent Assoc 1998;129:871–877.

15 Turksel Dulgergil C, Satici O, Yildirim I, Yavuz I: Prevention of caries in children by preventive and operative dental care for mothers in rural Anatolia, Turkey. Acta Odontol Scand 2004;62:251–257.

16 Nogueira RD, Alves AC, Napimoga MH, Smith DJ, Mattos-Graner RO: Characterization of salivary immunoglobulin A responses in children heavily exposed to the oral bacterium *Streptococcus mutans*: influence of specific antigen recognition in infection. Infect Immun 2005;73:5675–5684.

17 Psoter WJ, Zhang H, Pendrys DG, Morse DE, Mayne ST: Classification of dental caries patterns in the primary dentition: a multidimensional scaling analysis. Community Dent Oral Epidemiol 2003;31:231–238.

18 Johnsen DC, Bhat M, Kim MT, Hagman FT, Allee LM, Creedon RL, Easley MW: Caries levels and patterns in head start children in fluoridated and non-fluoridated, urban and non-urban sites in Ohio, USA. Community Dent Oral Epidemiol 1986;14:206–210.

19 Johnsen DC, Schubot D, Bhat M, Jones PK: Caries pattern identification in primary dentition: a comparison of clinician assignment and clinical analysis groupings. Pediatr Dent 1993;15:113–115.

20 Vanobbergen J, Lesaffre E, Garcia-Zattera MJ, Jara A, Martens L, Declerck D: Caries patterns in primary dentition in 3-, 5- and 7-year-old children: spatial correlation and preventive consequences. Caries Res 2007;41:16–25.

21 Saravanan S, Madivanan I, Subashini B, Felix JW: Prevalence pattern of dental caries in the primary dentition among school children. Ind J Dent Res 2005;16:140–146 (erratum published in Ind J Dent Res 2006;17:10).

22 Elfrink ME, Veerkamp JS, Kalsbeek H: Caries pattern in primary molars in Dutch 5-year-old children. Eur Arch Paediatr Dent 2006;7:236–240.

23 Wyne A, Darwish S, Adenubi J, Battata S, Khan N: The prevalence and pattern of nursing caries in Saudi preschool children. Int J Paediatr Dent 2001;11:361–364 (erratum published in Int J Paediatr Dent 2001;11:460).

24 Paul TR: Dental health status and caries pattern of preschool children in al-Kharj, Saudi Arabia. Saudi Med J 2003;24:1347–1351.

25 Poulsen VJ: Caries risk children in the Danish Child Dental Service. Scand J Primary Health Care 1987;5:169–175.

26 Warren JJ, Slayton RL, Yonezu T, Kanellis MJ, Levy SM: Interdental spacing and caries in the primary dentition. Pediatr Dent 2003;25:109–113.

27 Macek MD, Beltran-Aguilar ED, Lockwood SA, Malvitz DM: Updated comparison of the caries susceptibility of various morphological types of permanent teeth. J Public Health Dent 2003;63:174–182.

28 Selwitz RH, Winn DM, Kingman A, Zion GR: The prevalence of dental sealants in the US population: findings from NHANES III, 1988–1991. J Dent Res 1996;75(spec iss):652–660.

29 Mejare I, Kallestal C, Stenlund H, Johansson H: Caries development from 11 to 22 years of age: a prospective radiographic study. Prevalence and distribution. Caries Res 1998;32:10–16.

30 Psoter W, Gebrian B, Prophete S, Reid B, Katz R: Effect of early childhood malnutrition on tooth eruption in Haitian adolescents. Community Dent Oral Epidemiol 2008;36:179–189.

31 Alvarez JO: Nutrition, tooth development, and dental caries. Am J Clin Nutr 1995;61:410S-416S.

32 Greenwell AL, Johnsen D, Di Santis TA, Gerstenmaier J, Limbert N: Longitudinal evaluation of caries patterns from the primary to the mixed dentition. Pediatr Dent 1990;12:278–282.

33 Skeie MS, Raadal M, Strand GV, Espelid I: The relationship between caries in the primary dentition at 5 years of age and permanent dentition at 10 years of age – a longitudinal study. Int J Paediatr Dent 2006;16:152–160.

34 O'Sullivan DM, Tinanoff N: The association of early dental caries patterns with caries incidence in preschool children. J Public Health Dent 1996;56:81–83.

35 Nyvad B, Fejerskov O, Josephsen K: Organic structures of developmental origin in human surface enamel. Scand J Dent Res 1988;96:288–292.

36 Loesche WJ, Eklund S, Earnest R, Burt B: Longitudinal investigation of bacteriology of human fissure decay: epidemiological studies in molars shortly after eruption. Infect Immun 1984;46:765–772.

37 Carvalho JC, Ekstrand KR, Thylstrup A: Dental plaque and caries on occlusal surfaces of first permanent molars in relation to stage of eruption. J Dent Res 1989;68:773–779.

38 Carvalho JC, Ekstrand KR, Thylstrup A: Results after 1 year of non-operative occlusal caries treatment of erupting permanent first molars. Community Dent Oral Epidemiol 1991;19:23–28.

39 Ekstrand KR, Christiansen J, Christiansen ME: Time and duration of eruption of first and second permanent molars: a longitudinal investigation. Community Dent Oral Epidemiol 2003;31:344–350.

40 Ahmad N, Gelesko S, Shugars D, White RP Jr, Blakey G, Haug RH, Offenbacher S, Phillips C: Caries experience and periodontal pathology in erupting third molars. J Oral Maxillofac Surg 2008;66:948–953.

41 Shugars DA, Elter JR, Jacks MT, White RP, Phillips C, Haug RH, Blakey GH: Incidence of occlusal dental caries in asymptomatic third molars. J Oral Maxillofac Surg 2005;63:341–346.

42 Hopcraft MS, Morgan MV: Pattern of dental caries experience on tooth surfaces in an adult population. Community Dent Oral Epidemiol 2006;34:174–183.

43 Hannigan A, O'Mullane DM, Barry D, Schafer F, Roberts AJ: A caries susceptibility classification of tooth surfaces by survival time. Caries Res 2000;34:103–108.

44 Richardson PS, McIntyre IG: Susceptibility of tooth surfaces to carious attack in young adults. Community Dent Health 1996;13:163–168.

45 Chestnutt IG, Schafer F, Jacobson AP, Stephen KW: Incremental susceptibility of individual tooth surfaces to dental caries in Scottish adolescents. Community Dent Oral Epidemiol 1996;24:11–16.

46 McDonald SP, Sheiham A: The distribution of caries on different tooth surfaces at varying levels of caries – a compilation of data from 18 previous studies. Community Dent Health 1992;9:39–48.

47 Dummer PM, Oliver SJ, Hicks R, Kindon A, Addy M, Shaw WC: Factors influencing the initiation of carious lesions in specific tooth surfaces over a 4-year period in children between the ages of 11–12 years and 15–16 years. J Dent 1990;18:190–197.

48 Berman DS, Slack GL: Susceptibility of tooth surfaces to carious attack: a longitudinal study. Br Dent J 1973;134:135–139.

49 Carlos JP, Gittelsohn AM: Longitudinal studies of the natural history of caries. II. A life-table study of caries incidence in the permanent teeth. Arch Oral Biol 1965;10:739–751.

50 Barr JH, Diodati RR, Stephens RG: Incidence of caries at different locations on the teeth. J Dent Res 1957;36:536–545.

51 Mejare I, Stenlund H, Zelezny-Holmlund C: Caries incidence and lesion progression from adolescence to young adulthood: a prospective 15-year cohort study in Sweden. Caries Res 2004;38:130–141.

52 Stenlund H, Mejare I, Kallestal C: Caries incidence rates in Swedish adolescents and young adults with particular reference to adjacent approximal tooth surfaces: a methodological study. Community Dent Oral Epidemiol 2003;31:361–367.

53 Machiulskiene V, Nyvad B, Baelum V: Prevalence and severity of dental caries in 12-year-old children in Kaunas, Lithuania 1995. Caries Res 1998;32:175–180.

54 Mejare I, Kallest l C, Stenlund H: Incidence and progression of approximal caries from 11 to 22 years of age in Sweden: a prospective radiographic study. Caries Res 1999;33:93–100.

55 Shwartz M, Grondahl HG, Pliskin JS, Boffa J: A longitudinal analysis from bite-wing radiographs of the rate of progression of approximal carious lesions through human dental enamel. Arch Oral Biol 1984;29:529–536.

56 Mejare I, Stenlund H: Caries rates for the mesial surface of the first permanent molar and the distal surface of the second primary molar from 6 to 12 years of age in Sweden. Caries Res 2000;34:454–461.

57 Berkey CS, Douglass CW, Valachovic RW, Chauncey HH: Longitudinal radiographic analysis of carious lesion progression. Community Dent Oral Epidemiol 1988;16:83–90.

58 Warren JJ, Levy SM, Broffitt B, Kanellis MJ: Longitudinal study of non-cavitated carious lesion progression in the primary dentition. J Public Health Dent 2006;66:83–87.

59 McArdle LW, Renton TF: Distal cervical caries in the mandibular second molar: an indication for the prophylactic removal of the third molar? Br J Oral Maxillofac Surg 2006;44:42–45.

60 Mariri BP, Levy SM, Warren JJ, Bergus GR, Marshall TA, Broffitt B: Medically administered antibiotics, dietary habits, fluoride intake and dental caries experience in the primary dentition. Community Dent Oral Epidemiol 2003;31:40–51.

61 ten Cate JM: Remineralization of caries lesions extending into dentin. J Dent Res 2001;80:1407–1411.

62 Pitts NB, Renson CE: Monitoring the behaviour of posterior approximal carious lesions by image analysis of serial standardised bitewing radiographs. Br Dent J 1987;162:15–21.

63 Backer Dirks O: Posteruptive changes in dental enamel. J Dent Res 1966;45:503–511.

64 Fejerskov O, Nyvad B, Kidd EAM: Pathology of dental caries; in Fejerskov O, Kidd EAM (eds): Dental Caries: The Disease and Its Clinical Management, ed 2. Oxford, Blackwell Munksgaard, 2008, pp19–48.

65 Al-Khateeb S, Forsberg CM, de Josselin de Jong E, Angmar-Mansson B: A longitudinal laser fluorescence study of white spot lesions in orthodontic patients. Am J Orthod Dentofacial Orthop 1998;113:595–602.

66 Nyvad B, Machiulskiene V, Baelum V: Reliability of a new caries diagnostic system differentiating between active and inactive caries lesions. Caries Res 1999;33:252–260.

67 Koulourides T, Sims RM: Artificial caries studied with intermittent demineralizing and mineralizing treatments of teeth. Ala J Med Sci 1967;4:282–288.

Hafsteinn Eggertsson, DDS, MSD, PhD, Assistant Professor
Department of Preventive and Community Dentistry Oral Health Research Center
Indiana University School of Dentistry
415 Lansing Street
Indianapolis, IN 46202 (USA)
Tel. +1 317 274 8822, Fax +1 317 274 5425, E-Mail heggerts@iupui.edu

Assessing Patients' Health Behaviours

Essential Steps for Motivating Patients to Adopt and Maintain Behaviours Conducive to Oral Health

Ruth Freeman[a] · Amid Ismail[b]

[a]Oral Health and Health Research Programme, Dental Health Services Research Unit, University of Dundee, Dundee, UK; [b]Maurice H. Kornberg School of Dentistry, Temple University, Philadelphia, Pa., USA

Abstract

This chapter provides a summary of various approaches to behaviour change in oral health. The current research evidence does not support the practice of giving 'instructions' or 'advice' to patients as a means of modifying their attitudes or changing their health behaviours. A number of explanatory models are described which address both the complexity and the factors that influence and predict an individual's health behaviour. A practical guide of what should be assessed and professional assumptions which may be made to assist patients change and maintain their health behaviours are provided. The potential for difficulty during this assessment period is raised since this awareness will allow for flexibility when negotiating with patients to help them develop strategies to modify, change and maintain their health behaviours. Thus, the last part of the chapter describes new approaches that rely on multiple models that focus on patients' or recipients' beliefs, desired goals and readiness to change which are preferable to the traditional patient education approaches in dentistry.

Copyright © 2009 S. Karger AG, Basel

There is an assumption that changing people's behaviours is difficult and not attainable. Unfortunately this conclusion is based on employing oversimplified models for changing oral health behaviours. Dentists and dental hygienists have always assumed that their task is to provide appropriate and evidence-based health information, which increases *knowledge*, causes a modification in *attitudes* and subsequently a change in health *behaviour*. This educational model is known as the KAB model, and while it improves people's awareness of the causation of ill health it does little to change their health behaviours. Often people will appear to act in one way while still being aware of the ill effects their behaviour has upon their health. For Festinger [1] these patients are experiencing a cognitive dissonance – for clinicians it may seem that their patients are being awkward and difficult ignoring the professional advice which has been provided. The question, thus, enters the dentists' mind: 'How can I

Table 1. Components of the HBM [5]

Component	Definition of component
Perceived susceptibility	The individual's perceptions of getting ill
Perceived severity	The individual's perception of the seriousness of a condition and its health consequences
Perceived benefits	The individual's belief that the advised health action will reduce the seriousness of the disease
Perceived barriers	The perceived psychological, time and financial costs or barriers regarding compliance with the recommended actions
Cues to action	Readiness to act
Self-efficacy	Confidence to adopt the recommended behaviour

get the patient to change?' Another perspective on the reasons for this dissonance is that dental knowledge provided by oral health professionals is usually non-tailored to each patient's level of readiness to change, knowledge level, other concomitant life stressors and influencing events. In the current model for oral health education, the patient is assumed to be static. This chapter presents an introduction to different approaches to behavioural change to promote oral health. There is currently no single model that can be used exclusively in changing patients' behaviours. Rather, the best practice is to adopt or integrate aspects of different models that best fit the desired targeted behaviour and the population of interest.

Definition of Health Behaviours

Central to the clinician's dilemma is the understanding of what constitutes 'health behaviours'. According to Nutbeam [2] health behaviour is defined as 'any activity undertaken by an individual, regardless of actual or perceived health status, for the purpose of promoting, protecting or maintaining health, whether or not such behaviour is objectively effective towards that end'.

However, Nutbeam [2] voices caution and suggests that health behaviours must be distinguished from 'risk behaviours' which he defines as 'behaviours associated with increased susceptibility to a specific cause of ill health'. Therefore an examination of the literature does not provide a simple explanation of the term health behaviour. There is wide diversity among the various theoretical and explanatory models which are said to assist in the understanding of health and its associated behaviours. Why should it be necessary to conceptualize health and its associated behaviours as complex and interactive cognitive models? Surely a simple definition – such as 'the actions associated with health' would be enough to understand health behaviours and to promote oral health interventions for the maintenance of health? To support this view would be to ignore the complexities of health behaviours – and the influences both internal and external – to the individual which affect health and its associated behaviours.

Stepwise Model to Assess Oral Health Behaviours

In order to assist the patient to adopt behaviours conducive to health it is necessary to conceptualize the assessment of a patient's health behaviour as a series of steps. Hence it is necessary for dental health professionals to be familiar with [1] models of behaviour and perceptions of need, [2] what should be assessed and as models of behaviour change and methods to assess the patient's readiness to change [3].

Step 1: Understanding Behaviour – Models of Behaviour and Perceptions of Need

A number of explanatory cognitive models exist which predict and illustrate the complexity of health behaviours. In this section models of behaviour will be described in order to demonstrate, first, the complexity of health behaviours and, second, how factors internal and external to the individuals impact upon their health behaviours.

The Health Belief Model
The first of these is the 'health belief model' (HBM) developed by Hochbaum [3] and Rosenstock [4]. The HBM is based on the premise that if an individual believes him/herself to be susceptible to an illness, that the illness has significant health impacts and that the perceived benefits outweigh the perceived barriers of taking actions to support health, then the individual will adopt behaviours conducive to health (table 1).

Figure 1 shows the basic components of the model and also illustrates 'cues for action' such as for example 'oral cancer awareness week' as well as 'modifying factors' such as age, confidence (self-efficacy) or health knowledge. The HBM has been criticized with regard to its ability to predict the adoption of behaviours conducive to health; nevertheless, the HBM has been shown to be of value in the prediction of toothbrushing behaviours in childhood with perceived susceptibility being the strongest predictor of preventive health behaviours [6].

The HBM only focusses on individual perception, modifying factors and perceived benefits in determining behaviour change. Given that each individual has to determine whether they need to change and when and how to change, attempts to increase knowledge or perception of susceptibility and potential benefits, like the KAB model, cannot alone lead to significant change in behaviour without considering the enabling and modifying factors that influence an individual to behave in a certain way for a lifetime. A systematic review concluded that the HBM impact on changing behaviour is inconsistent because the model focusses only on predisposing factors. New models were proposed that address this limitation.

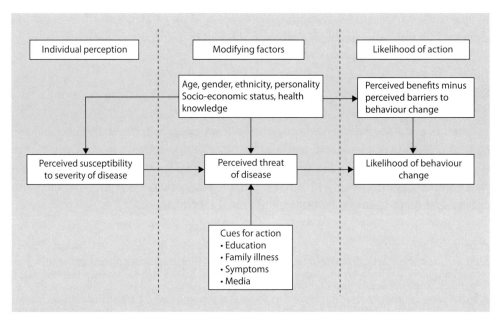

Fig. 1. The HBM [5].

A systematic, quantitative review of studies that had applied the HBM among adults into the late 1980s found it lacking in consistent predictive power for many behaviours, probably because its scope is limited to predisposing factors [7]. One study that specifically compared its predictive power with other models found that it accounted for a smaller proportion of the variance in diet, exercise and smoking behaviours than did the theory of reasoned action, theory of planned behaviour and the precede-proceed model [8].

The Theory of Planned Behaviour
The theory of planned behaviour (TPB) conceptualized by Ajzen [9] defines behaviour in terms of volition and intention to act. This explanatory model is based on the premise that people make use of all the available information in order to perform or not perform a particular behaviour. In the TPB, the role of attitudes and the evaluation of those attitudes together with the attitudes of important others and motivation to comply with their wishes (the so-called subjective norm) are said to be predictive of the intention to perform a particular behaviour. In addition, the TPB recognizes the importance of 'perceived behavioural control' which is a combination of control beliefs and perceived power. Therefore, the importance of confidence or self-efficacy is pivotal in the prediction of an individual's intention to perform or not to perform a particular behaviour. It is important to consider the TPB when trying to understand health behaviours because it takes into account factors internal to the individual such

as attitudes and perceived behavioural control as well as external factors such as the role of significant others. In the TPB these influences are appreciated as being central in the prediction of behaviour.

The Self-Determination Theory
The self-determination theory [10–12] has often been considered as providing a strong theoretical framework within which to understand how to change behaviours. Deci and Ryan and their group [10–12] proposed that behaviour changes motivated by intrinsic factors (e.g. inherently novel, enjoyable, stimulating, self-driven and satisfying) are more sustainable than those produced by extrinsic factors (e.g. coercion, external reward or fear) as well as those that are amotivational. New behaviour change approaches build intrinsic motivation in a way that longer, more confrontational, educational or skill-focussed interventions may not. These client-centred approaches allow for *value linkage* between an individual's personal values and the behaviours he/she chooses.

Self-Efficacy Theory
According to Bandura [13–15], self-efficacy is the 'belief in one's effectiveness in performing specific tasks'. Self-efficacious individuals are more likely to adopt behaviours compared with those with low self-efficacy. Self-efficacy is a complex state that cannot be easily taught; rather it is developed by understanding social, cognitive and environmental factors that influence the desire to achieve an outcome. Self-efficacy is a key factor for achieving a state of change or adopting behaviours. Self-determination can only be achieved through self-reflection on personal beliefs and self-evaluation of priorities and experiences. Self-reflection and self-evaluation increase the chance that an individual will take actions to attain performance skills. The self-efficacy theory portends that in order to initiate action, humans need to define their desired outcomes and then navigate through their inner thoughts and paradoxes to take steps to achieve them.

Health-Directed and Health-Related Behaviours and Concepts of Need
Early work conducted by Smith [16] examined the toothbrushing behaviours of 12- to 17-year-old adolescents in order to understand preventive health behaviours. Her findings suggested that the majority of girls did not feel susceptible to periodontal disease nor did they regard it as a threat to their oral health. Although the girls brushed their teeth daily, they did not consider toothbrushing as a means of prevention and did not identify bleeding gums as a cue for health action. It seemed that the girls' toothbrushing activity was associated with grooming rather than the prevention of gingivitis. Toothbrushing in this scenario was a health-related rather than a health-directed behaviour.

When considering explanatory models of health behaviours, it is of value to reflect upon the concepts of health-related and health-directed behaviours. In essence health-directed behaviours are those which are performed by an individual primarily to prevent disease whereas health-related behaviours are those actions which are primarily performed to improve, for example, self-esteem but where there is a secondary 'spin-off' for health. A good example is the reduction in frequency of sugar consumption: some people will reduce their sugar consumption to prevent dental caries (health-directed behaviour) whereas others will reduce their sugar consumption to look better (health-related behaviour) which will have the added benefits of improving oral health and reducing obesity.

Integral to health-directed and health-related behaviours is the individual's perceptions of his/her health needs. Ong [17] has suggested that people's health care needs are traded off against other more urgent or important needs such as family illness or socio-economic status. Therefore oral health education goals will be different for different people. If dental professionals wish their patients to adopt more healthy behaviours, they must consider the specific health 'needs' of their patient(s). Bradshaw [18] has identified 3 different categories of health needs:

(1) *normative need* is a professionally defined need; it is identified by health professionals, when they diagnose disease or perceive a fall in acceptable standards; it is dictated by professional training and is often based on value judgements;

(2) *felt need* is what people feel about their health needs; this is a lay perception of health needs; it is what patients want and what they think needs to be done; this is often different from professionally defined need and may cause conflict between clinician and patient;

(3) *expressed need* is the need that people vocalize – in words and actions; these are different from felt needs which the patient may feel but be unable to verbalize to the clinician.

Step 2: What Should Be Assessed and Professional Assumptions

The first step in the formulation of the patient health behaviour assessment has examined several models of behaviour. These models illustrated the complexity of factors internal and external to the individual which were predictive of behaviour. The role of attitudes and self-efficacy is central in explaining the adoption of a particular behaviour while the role of external factors – such as family members – is salient in predicting behaviour. There are, therefore, various internal and external factors which must be considered when providing one-to-one oral health education. As these influences also include patient perceptions of health-directed behaviours, health-related behaviours and health needs, it is necessary as the second step in the patient behavioural assessment to:
- assess the patient's level of understanding of the disease condition, severity or behaviour;
- assess the patient's level of oral health knowledge;

- ask the patient about his/her previous compliance with oral health advice;
- assess the patient's ability for self-care;
- assess the patient's attitudes towards oral health;
- ask the patient about the oral health experiences of his/her family, peers and community;
- ask the patient about the attitudes towards oral health of his/her family, peers and community.

Once the patient's details have been obtained, patient and health professional enter a new phase. Often in this phase the health professional may feel that the time has come for the patient to change and adopt a raft of new behaviours conducive to health. This is a *dangerous time* as the health professional may impose oral health information upon the patient in the belief that the patient [19–21]: (1) is ready for change, (2) should change now, and (3) that dental health is his/her prime motivating factor.

When this approach fails, the health professionals may feel that: (1) their position as a health professional had been usurped, (2) the tenor of their approach was incorrect, and (3) the consultation had failed.

The above are dangerous assumptions and do not allow for flexibility in the process of change [19–21]. The danger for both clinician and patient is that the encounter will be perceived as a difficult interaction with fears that an impasse has been reached. However, this is not the case and the next step in the process is to understand the patient's behaviour and how the patient's feelings and opinions may influence and can be used as an agent for change in the adoption and maintenance of behaviours conducive to health.

Step 3: Understanding Behaviour Change – Motivational Interviewing and Transtheoretical Model

Thus, at the centre of any behavioural strategy to assist the patient adopt and maintain behaviours conducive to health is the requirement to incorporate patient information into a preventive plan which enables change. Various models of health behaviour change exist, in this regard. They range from clinician-centred to patient- or client-centred strategies. Table 2 illustrates these models as a continuum from being clinician to client centred. The first model is the educational model or the KAB model which relies upon the health professional providing health education to explore attitudes in order to change health behaviours. Similarly, the behaviour change model relies on the clinician providing information to change behaviour by negotiating and setting health goals to enable shifts in behaviour over time. The final model is the client-centred model. This model takes into account the influences or factors which both inhibit and enable the patient to change. Hence the health professional follows the patient's lead by recognizing the patient's abilities and difficulties when attempting to adopt behaviours conducive to health.

Table 2. Models of health education to promote behaviour change [22, 23]

Model of health education	Aim	Health education/ promotion activity	Examples for primary dental care
Education or KAB model	To provide health knowledge and understanding; health decisions are made and acted upon	Health education given together with an exploration of attitudes; skills are provided for healthier living	Smoking cessation programmes in dental practice
Behaviour change model	To change health behaviours and improve health	Assist attitude and behaviour changes to encourage shifts from unhealthy to healthier behaviours	One-to-one dental health education at the chair side on dietary advice for prevention of dental caries
Client-centred models (self-determination, self-efficacy, TTM)	To negotiate health goals from the patient's felt and expressed needs	Patients set the agenda and decide which health issues should be discussed; patients are empowered to negotiate their identified health goals	Negotiation of oral health goals to assist adolescents to reduce consumption of acidic drinks

In order to assist the patient in complying and maintaining newly adopted behaviours the health professionals must integrate what they know about the patients' level of understanding of health-related attitudes, including difficulties in self-care and the readiness to change. This awareness on the part of the health professional counteracts the fear that an impasse has been reached. In essence the health professional follows the patient's lead and in doing so adopts the elements of good practice when negotiating behaviour change [19–21]: (1) respect for the autonomy of the patients and that their choices are important; (2) readiness to change must be taken into account; (3) ambivalence is common, and reasons for it need to be explored and understood; (4) targets/goals should be identified by the patients; (5) the expert (you) provides information and support, and (6) the patient is the active decision-maker.

Motivational Interviewing
Motivational interviewing incorporates all the elements of good practice [19, 20] and is based on the patients setting their own agenda of change, and thus integral to motivational interviewing is the patient's readiness to change. These are the central tenets of motivational interviewing as the dental professional negotiates her/his way through the motivational pathway. Figure 2 is a schematic of motivational interviewing. The schema is divided up into phases in order to present an overview of motivational interviewing. The first phase of the procedure is to decide upon which

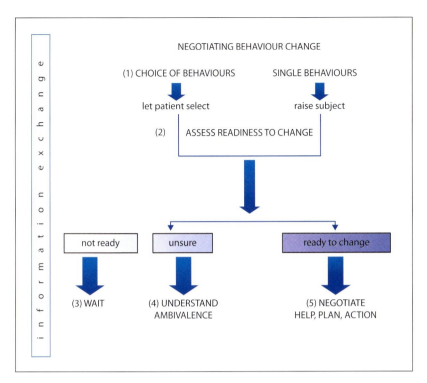

Fig. 2. Motivational interviewing.

behaviour to change; the second phase is to access the patients' readiness to change and the third phase is to act upon the patient's state of readiness to change. In motivational interviewing, the dentists or dental hygienists neither provide direct advice nor suggest what the patients should do. The primary goal of the process of motivational interviewing is to assist patients to make their own decisions and set their preferred goals. The application of motivational interviewing requires developing new communication skills such as different levels of reflection, asking open questions, rolling with the resistance, discovering ambivalence and engaging patients in change talk.

Phase 1: Which Behaviour to Change?

The patient may have one or several oral health problems which could be helped by changing and adopting behaviours conducive to oral health. In the situation where there is just one behaviour – for example the use of interdental cleaning – the dental health professional may raise the subject. When there are many behaviours, the use of the agenda-setting chart (fig. 3) provides the patients with an opportunity to choose which behaviour they would like to change. In figure 3 the example provided is improving periodontal health. The behaviours that the patient may choose range

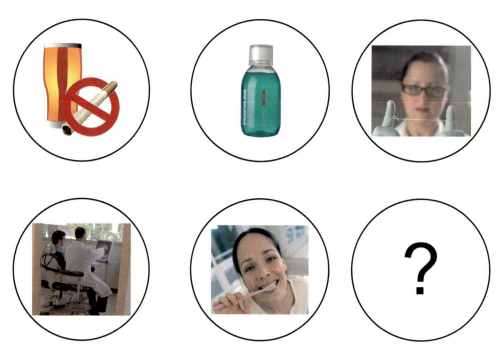

Fig. 3. Agenda-setting chart.

from smoking cessation to toothbrushing. In addition there is a 'query' for the patient to bring his/her own suggestion for change.

Phase 2: Readiness to Change?
Together the dental health professional and the patient must decide on the patient's degree of ambivalence or 'readiness to change'. This may be done in several ways, and two examples are provided here. First, there is a readiness rule in which the patient indicates on a sliding scale from 'not ready' through 'unsure' to 'ready' his/her readiness to change. Alternatively, the patient may examine the pros and cons of changing oral health behaviours using a 'balance sheet' (fig. 4). The ensuing discussion between the dental professional and patient allows an assessment of the patient's readiness to change to be made (fig. 4). Irrespective of which method is used to assess readiness to change, what is essential is that patients are involved in identifying their own degree of ambivalence and the behaviours to be modified.

Phases 3–5: Not Ready, Ambivalent and Ready to Change
There are 3 possible outcomes of motivational interviewing:
  in phase 3, the patient is not ready; this must be accepted, and the dental health professional must wait;

	No change	Change
	Costs Feel unattractive Diffecult to smile Difficult to kiss partner	Costs Will upset my routines Willl take too much time Dental treatment cost too much
	Benefits Feel self-conscious	Benefits Increased self-esteem

Fig. 4. The balance sheet to assess ambivalence.

in phase 4, the patient is ambivalent; the indecision of the patient must be acknowledged, and the dentist must try to understand the patient's resistances to change;

in phase 5, the patient is ready to change, i.e. the oral health behaviour has been identified and the oral health goals negotiated.

The use of health-negotiating goal agendae such as Be SMART – be specific, measurable, attainable, realistic and time-related – may be used to devise specific oral health goals which the patient will be able to attain within a time period. At this time, the support from the health professional is essential.

Motivational interviewing has been used in dentistry to assist patients to change their oral health behaviours. In Britain [24] and in North America [25, 26], client-centred approaches have been used to increase awareness, modify attitudes and promote oral health. In the work conducted by Weinstein et al. [25, 26], they used the vehicle of oral health to promote 'self-efficacy' and the 'patient's competence'. Details are provided as to how the dental health professional 'provides advice... and emphasizes patient choice'.

Perhaps what is of central importance is how the dental professional will cope with patient ambivalence or resistance to change and how the dentist's responses will affect the patient's ability to adopt and maintain behaviours conducive to oral health: 'Useful strategies, for example, are to emphasize choice, avoid arguing or even agree with the patient, saying that he or she has a valid point' [25].

In essence the dental health professional enables the patient to maintain the treatment alliance [27] and to accept the oral health care which is being offered and provided. This is achieved by promoting rapport and understanding while reducing the likelihood of the patient feeling blamed and/or humiliated. The result of adopting a motivational interviewing approach was a reduction of 46% in obvious decay experience in young children whose parents had received the motivational interviewing intervention [28].

Transtheoretical Model of Behaviour Change
The transtheoretical model (TTM) of behaviour change is closely related to motivational interviewing [29]. The TTM is another client-centred strategy which

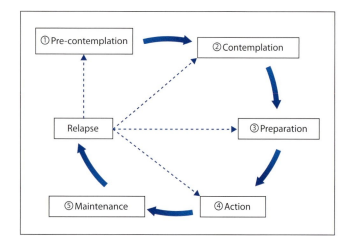

Fig. 5. The TTM of behaviour change.

acknowledges that behaviour change is a complex process. It is also dependent on the patient's ability to change and acknowledges that the patient's degree of ambivalence is of central importance. The role of the dental health professional is once more to identify the patients' state of readiness to change and to provide help and support to enable them to change from less healthy to healthier actions. For the patient who is ambivalent, the stages-of-change model provides a solution to assist the patient move from being a 'chronic contemplator' to getting ready for 'action'. In this model, change is seen as a process, which has 5 interlinking stages. Figure 5 shows the various phases of the model which are described separately in order to present an overview of the TTM.

The TTM stages of change start with precontemplation and take the dental health professional and patient on a road through contemplation, preparation, action to maintenance and the possibility of relapse at every stage of the journey.

Precontemplation
The patient moves from being unaware to being aware of the need to change. It is at this stage that motivational interviewing is used to assess ambivalence and readiness to change. The discussion of the benefits ('the pros') and the barriers ('the cons') provides the basis of the precontemplation stage. Interventions used include providing patients with health information and discovering lifestyle problems which might act as barriers to progressing to the next stage.

Contemplation
Patients are weighing up the benefits ('the pros') against the barriers ('the cons') of adopting behaviours conducive to oral health. These patients are not yet ready to change. Often patients may seem 'stuck' in the contemplation stage and become 'chronic contemplators'. In order to assist these ambivalent patients, they should be

seen frequently and supported to enable the promotion of self-efficacy, confidence and eventual preparation for behaviour change.

Preparation

This phase may take a long time. It is an essential phase for chronic contemplators as preparation time will allow the time for concerns and anxieties to be discussed which has the effect to reduce ambivalence while improving self-awareness and self-image. The clinician's task is to provide patients with information and to assist them to think about their worries, difficulties and feelings about changing.

Action and Maintenance

As patients enter these phases, they have resolved their conflict or ambivalence. The pros of changing now outweigh the cons. During the action phase the dental health professional works with patients and using such strategies for goal setting as Be SMART assists them to identify realistic oral health goals. In the maintenance phase, the interventions are shorter but more intensive and more participative to support patients maintain their newly acquired oral health behaviour.

Relapse

Relapse is common and occurs when unhealthy behaviours are reinstated. Nevertheless this provides time to re-examine and renegotiate oral health goals and to recognize what has been achieved and what will be achieved again. During the relapse phase the dental health professional must be supportive. The patient must be assisted to identify more realistic and achievable goals. After the relapse phase, patients do not return to precontemplation but may return to the contemplation stage where they may progress quickly through preparation to action.

The TTM stages of change have been used to promote healthier diets [30], changing oral hygiene behaviours [31, 32] and enable periodontal patients to enter smoking cessation programmes [33].

An essential part of the TTM stages of change is the assessment of the patients' stage of change which may be assessed using a questionnaire developed by Prochaska et al. [34]. This inventory consists of 20 questions which are of 5-point scale format. The 20 questions reflect the processes of change. The questions illustrate the means by which people change their behaviours. There are 10 processes of change questions which are related to, for example, 'the pros and cons' of changing, self-efficacy or confidence which predict movement through the various stages of change.

Tilliss et al. [32] developed a 4-item questionnaire to determine the patient's degree of readiness to change regarding interdental cleaning. Entitled the Stages of Change Instrument, the questionnaire described interdental cleaning and asked about the frequency and intention to clean interdentally. The accompanying legend allowed the dental health professional to place the patients at the correct stage that relates to their awareness and preparation to take action to change. The dental professional, together with the patient, can now devise an oral health intervention appropriate to the patient's position on the TTM stages of change to enable the patient adopt and maintain behaviours conducive to oral health.

Final Steps and Conclusions

In order to bring about lasting and effective changes in behaviours conducive to health, oral health clinicians must help patients explore their oral health attitudes, uncover their health values and encourage them to identify their own oral health agenda. This involves the dental health professional providing support for the patient and adopting a patient-centred approach. In this chapter a number of health behaviour and health behaviour change models have been presented to demonstrate the complexity of helping patients adopt and maintain new behaviours conducive to oral health. Moreover advice has been given regarding how these models may be used in the dental setting to enable health behaviour change.

This introductory chapter, thus, presented a summary of approaches to behavioural change in oral health. The practice of giving 'instructions' or 'advice' to patients is no longer supported by current evidence on approaches to modify health behaviours. New approaches that rely on multiple models that focus on patients' or recipients' beliefs, desired goals and readiness to change are preferable to the traditional patient education approaches in dentistry. The emergence of interactive web-based programs can aid in developing useful tools for practitioners.

References

1 Festinger L: A Theory of Cognitive Dissonance. Stanford, Stanford University Press, 1957.
2 Nutbeam D: Health promotion glossary. Health Promot Int 1998;13:349–364.
3 Hochbaum GM: Public participation in medical screening programs; a sociopsychological study. PHS Publication No 572. Washington, Government Printing Office, 1958.
4 Rosenstock IM: The health belief model and preventive health behaviour. Health Educ Monogr 1974;2:354–386.
5 Janz NK, Champion VL, Strecher VJ: The health belief model; in Glanz K, Rimer BK, Lewis FM (eds): Health Behaviour and Health Education: Theory, Research and Practice, ed 3. San Francisco, Jossy-Bass, 2002.
6 Pine CM, McGoldrick PM, Burnside G, Curnow MM, Chesters RK, Nicholson J, Huntington E: An intervention programme to establish regular toothbrushing: understanding parents' beliefs and motivating children. Int Dent J Suppl 2000;50: 312–323.
7 Harrison JA, Mullen PD, Green LW: A meta-analysis of studies of the health belief model. Health Educ Res 1992;7:107–116.
8 Mullen PD, Hersey JC, Iverson DC: Health behaviour models compared. Soc Sci Med 1987;24:973–981.
9 Ajzen I: The theory of planned behaviour. Org Behav Hum Decision Process 1991;50:179–211.
10 Deci EL, Koestner R, Ryan RM: A meta-analytic review of experiments examining the effects of extrinsic rewards on intrinsic motivation. Psychol Bull 1999;125:627–668.
11 Ryan RM, Kuhl J, Deci EL: Nature and autonomy: an organizational view of social and neurobiological aspects of self-regulation in behavior and development. Dev Psychopathol 1997;9:701–728.
12 Deci EL, Ryan RM: Intrinsic Motivation and Self-Determination in Human Behavior. New York, Plenum Press, 1985.
13 Bandura A: Reflections on self-efficacy. Adv Behav Res Ther 1978;1:237–269.

14 Bandura A: The self system in reciprocal determinism. Am Psychologist 1978;33:344–358.
15 Bandura A: Perceived self-efficacy in cognitive development and functioning. Educ Psychol 1993;28:117–148.
16 Smith JM: An evaluation of the applicability of the Rosenstock-Hochbaum health behaviour model to the prevention of periodontal disease in English schoolgirls. J Clin Periodontol 1974;1:222–231.
17 Ong BN: The Practice of Health Services Research. London, Chapman & Hall, 1993
18 Bradshaw J: The concept of human need. New Soc 1972;30:640–643.
19 Rollnick S, Mason P, Butler C: Health Behaviour Change: A Guide for Practitioners. Edinburgh, Churchill Livingstone, 1999.
20 Rollnick S, Kinnersley P, Stott N: Methods of helping patients with behaviour change. Br Med J 1993;307:188–190.
21 Rollnick S, Butler CC, McCambridge J, Kinnersley P, Elwyn G, Resnicow K: Consultations about changing behaviour. Br Med J 2005;331:961–963.
22 Burke FTJ, Freeman R: Preparing for Dental Practice. Oxford, Oxford University Press, 2004.
23 Freeman R, Humphris GM: Communicating in Dental Practice: Stress Free Dentistry and Improved Patient Care. London, Quintessence Publishing, 2006.
24 Blinkhorn AS, Gratix PJ, Holloway PJ, Wainright-Stringer YM, Warrd SJ, Worthington HV: A clustered randomised controlled trial of the value of dental health educators in general dental practice. Br Dent J 2003;195:395–400.
25 Weinstein P, Harrison R, Benton T: Motivating parents to prevent caries in their young children: one-year findings. J Am Dent Assoc 2004;135:731–737.
26 Weinstein P, Harrison R, Benton T: Motivating parents to prevent caries: confirming the beneficial effects of counselling. J Am Dent Assoc 2006;135:789–793.
27 Freeman R: Strategies for motivating the non-compliant patient. Br Dent J 1999;187:307–312.
28 Harrison R, Benton T, Everson-Stewart S, Weinstein P: Effect of motivational interviewing on rates of early childhood caries: a randomized trial. Pediatr Dent 2007;29:16–22.
29 Prochaska J, Di Clemente C: Toward a comprehensive model of change; in Millar W, Heather N (eds): Treating Addictive Behaviours: Process of Change. New York, Plenum Press, 1986.
30 Buchanan H, Coulson NS: Consumption of carbonated drinks in adolescents: a transtheoretical analysis. Child Care Health Dev 2006;4:441–447.
31 Kasila K, Poskiparta M, Kettunen T, Pietilä I: Oral health counselling in changing schoolchildren's oral hygiene habits: a qualitative study. Community Dent Oral Epidemiol 2006;34:419–428.
32 Tilliss TSI, Stach DJ, Cross-Poline GN, Annan SD, Astroth DB, Wolfe P: The transtheoretical model applied to an oral self-care behavioral change: development and testing of instruments for stages of change and decisional balance. J Dent Hyg 2003;77:16–26.
33 Martinelli E, Palmer RM, Wilson RF, Newton JT: Smoking behaviour and attitudes to periodontal health and quit smoking in patients with periodontal disease. J Clin Periodontol 2008;35:944–954.
34 Prochaska JO, Velicer WF, Di Clemente C, Fava JL: Measuring processes to change: applications to the cessation of smoking. J Consult Clin Psychol 1988;56:520–528.

Dr. Ruth Freeman
Dental Health Services Research Unit, Mackenzie Building
Kirsty Semple Way
Dundee DD2 4BF (UK)
Tel. +44 1382 420050, Fax +44 1382 420051, E-Mail r.e.freeman@chs.dundee.ac.uk

Personalized Treatment Planning

N.B. Pitts[a] · D. Richards[b], for the International Caries Detection and Assessment System Committee

[a]Dental Health Services and Research Unit, University of Dundee, Dundee, [b]Department of Public Health, NHS Forth Valley, Stirling, UK

Abstract

This chapter aims to outline a flexible framework which the dental team can use to bring together key elements of information about their patients and their patients' teeth in order to plan appropriate, patient-centred, caries management based on the application of best current evidence and practice. This framework can be enabled by the use of the International Caries Detection and Assessment System (ICDAS) clinical visual scoring systems for caries detection and activity, but also needs additional information about lesions and the patient to plan and then monitor the effectiveness of personalized caries care. The treatment planning process has evolved from restorative treatment decisions being largely made during clinical assessment as an examination of wet teeth proceeds, with limited charting and a minor role for patient factors. Best practice now involves a comprehensive examination being made systematically of clean dry teeth using sharp eyes and blunt probes. The ICDAS-enabled framework provides for information to be collected at the *tooth/surface level* (clinical visual lesion detection, lesion detection aids and lesion activity assessment) and at the *patient level* (patient caries risk assessment, dentition and lesion history and patient behavioural assessment). This information is then synthesized to inform *integrated, personalized treatment planning* which involves the choice of appropriate *treatment options* (background level care, preventive treatment options, operative treatment options) and then *recall, reassessment and monitoring*. Examples of international moves towards using integrated, personalized treatment planning for caries control are given, drawing on experiences in the UK, the USA and from the ICDAS Committee.

Copyright © 2009 S. Karger AG, Basel

This chapter aims to outline a flexible framework within which dentists and the dental team can bring together key elements of information about their patients and the condition of patients' teeth in order to plan appropriate, patient-centred caries management based on the application of best current evidence. This is a challenge as, in some areas, evidence is strong and conclusive – but in others high-quality research focussed on the clinical issues of concern has yet to be carried out and reported. As much of traditional practice in this area is also deficient in supporting evidence, the profession has to be guided by international consensus and expert opinion while research is carried out and synthesized over the longer term.

This framework can be enabled by the use of the International Caries Detection and Assessment System (ICDAS) clinical visual scoring systems for caries and has been developed by the ICDAS Committee as an open system built on a consensus around the best available evidence over a period of some years [1].

The shared vision of the ICDAS Committee is that:
- the ICDAS is developed and maintained as a clinical visual scoring system for use in clinical practice, research, epidemiology and dental education;
- the ICDAS achieves what it is designed to do, i.e. to lead to better-quality information to inform decisions about appropriate diagnosis, prognosis and clinical management at both the individual and public health levels;
- the ICDAS provides a framework to support and enable personalized comprehensive caries management for improved long-term health outcomes.

The focus of this chapter is around the second and third objectives, enabling integrated, personalized treatment planning at the individual patient level. This is enabled by clinical visual lesion detection and assessment, but also needs additional information about lesions and the patient to plan and then monitor the effectiveness of personalized caries care.

Evolution of the Treatment Planning Process for Caries

Figure 1 shows a schematic outline of a 'traditional' caries management approach from the typical practice in some countries of some decades ago. The teeth and tooth surfaces are examined; this was (and in some cases still is) often done with limited cleaning, with limited saliva control and with the use of a sharp explorer (probe). Treatment decisions are largely made on the basis of this clinical assessment as examination proceeds. Often, all that is recorded on a dental chart is the number of surfaces to be involved in any operative treatment deemed to be needed. Patient factors may play only a small part in the clinical decision-making process. The emphasis was on restoring (rather than extracting) teeth in an efficient way. As many examinations and treatment plans are carried out over months and years, this process becomes highly scripted in the head of the dentist and becomes almost 'automatic' [2]. Some of the diagnostic and prognostic steps originally in clinical decision-making can become lost in this scripted process. In some countries, this traditional model has been considered outdated for many years, in others it is still in use today, despite the well-known limitations of restorative-only treatment [3].

Figure 2 shows the outline of the contemporary ICDAS-enabled, patient-centred, caries management framework. This builds on the previous model, but there are now more specific areas that are considered, and examination is made systematically on clean dry teeth using sharp eyes and (generally) blunt probes applied with little force. The other chapters in this book provide the detail within each element of the framework and present the current understanding, evidence and position in each of the respective fields.

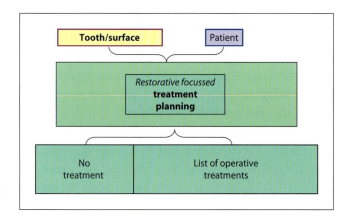

Fig. 1. Flow diagram for traditional caries management.

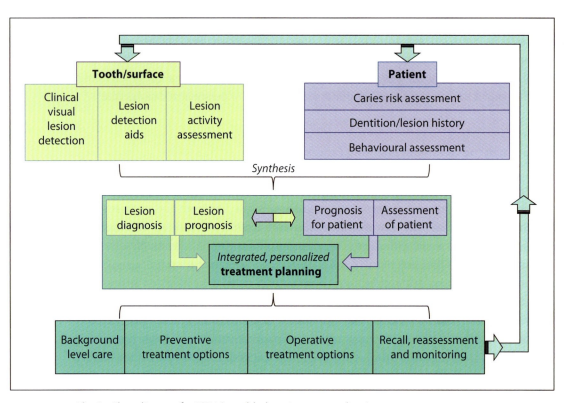

Fig. 2. Flow diagram for ICDAS-enabled, patient-centred caries management.

It is important however not to become lost in the potential complexity of these elements and their interactions. The intention is merely to provide a structure to enable the clinician to take into account all the necessary information required to plan treatment that is appropriate to the needs and wants of his or her patient. Individual dentists and groups will find efficient ways to operationalize this framework. The use of information technology, practice-based electronic patient records and clinical decision support tools may all help to smooth the way in which the framework can best be delivered efficiently in dental practices. Many dental teams and dental teaching institutions, particularly in Scandinavia and more recently Australia [4], advocate and use much of this information as they move to implement the type of *minimal intervention dentistry* advocated by the Fédération Dentaire Internationale in 2000 [5]. Across Europe this type of caries information has also been recognized as one of the priority oral heath indicators to be collected in the general practice setting [6, 7].

The focus in health care is shifting and evolving towards a more evidence-based and evidence-informed model where a pro-active, preventive stance is taken in order to control diseases and promote health effectively in a holistic way by using early detection of disease and planning treatment and care in the longer term over the life course. Caries management should embrace and be improved by these wider developments. The extent to which different groups of dentists and countries have moved from operative to non-operative/preventive treatment of dental caries in clinical practice is very variable but is an accelerating trend globally [8].

Figure 2 shows that the framework provides for information to be collected:
at the *tooth/surface level* by:
- clinical visual lesion detection [this vol., pp. 15–41];
- lesion detection aids, both conventional [this vol., pp. 42–51] and novel [this vol., pp. 52–62];
- lesion activity assessment [this vol., pp. 63–90];

at the *patient level* on:
- patient caries risk assessment [this vol., pp. 91–101];
- dentition and lesion history [this vol., pp. 102–112];
- patient behavioural assessment [this vol., pp. 113–127].

This information is then synthesized to inform personalized treatment planning (this chapter).

Integrated, personalized treatment planning involves selecting the choice of appropriate treatment options at multiple sites and setting up individualized recall/monitoring. This involves the planning of:
- background level care [this vol., pp. 144–148];
- preventive treatment options, traditional [this vol., pp. 149–155] and novel [this vol., pp. 156–163];
- operative treatment options, traditional [this vol., pp. 164–173] and novel [this vol., pp. 174–187];
- recall, reassessment and monitoring [this vol., pp. 188–198].

The challenges and opportunities associated with the *implementation* of this approach and framework to improving the detection, assessment, diagnosis and monitoring of caries in order to ensure optimal personalized caries management are many [see the chapter by Pitts, this vol., pp. 199–208]. It is also important to ensure consistency and clarity about the use of terminology in this area; otherwise, communications across dental interests and with other stakeholders are seriously impaired. The international consensus definitions set out in a glossary of key terms [see the chapter by Longbottom et al., this vol., pp. 209–216] can help avoid difficulties in this area.

The Importance of the Treatment Planning Process for Caries and Trends

Typically, the treatment planning process for caries receives comparatively little attention in dentistry; it is almost 'taken for granted' as dentists and dental organizations focus on more complex and 'high-tech' dental interventions. However, as the lifelong burden of caries care continues to be significant in personal, societal and economic terms, the clinical and patient information required as the foundation for planning effective care should be based on updated, comprehensive and relevant records about the disease and its status in the individual patient.

The international moves towards patient-centred care, which can have important benefits for attracting and retaining patients at the practice level, call for the information collected in this framework to be synthesized and the planned treatment options tailored for the individual patient. Consideration is given to patient circumstances and preferences, as well as to the dental team, health system and country contexts. Treatment plans are encouraged to be holistic, long term and flexible, with treatment options being chosen on the basis of best evidence and professional consensus. These plans are then implemented as shared care between the patient and an oral health team appropriate to the local setting. The dental team should take note of and make use of well-constructed guidelines and guidance in order to keep up to date as new evidence emerges. Changing professional responsibilities within the dental team and shifting medicolegal responsibilities should also be taken into consideration as these evolve and develop in many parts of the world.

Examples of Moving towards Integrated, Personalized Treatment Planning for Caries

UK Developments

Over the last decade there have been a number of parallel developments in the UK, from both the National Health Service (NHS) and the profession, which are gradually advancing record keeping, a preventive treatment philosophy for caries and individualized risk-based recalls for patients attending general practices.

In 2001 the Faculty of General Dental Practice published guidelines for clinical examination and record keeping [9] which set out the need for systematic and comprehensive information capture. Around this time there were radical discussions about the best way to provide modern, preventively focussed, effective care in NHS general practice under an initiative known as 'options for change' [10]. Although the subsequent implementation of payment arrangements in England and Wales to support this approach has proved problematic, there is now a clear focus on delivering caries prevention in practice [11]. In Scotland there has been a long-running focus on caries prevention, with national evidence-based guidance on the subject [12, 13].

In 2004, the National Institute for Clinical Excellence issued the formal guidance on 'Dental recall – recall interval between routine dental examinations' [14], which reviewed the evidence across all of oral health and recommended an individualized recall interval on the basis of the dentist's judgement, informed by integrating a number of risk factors. Further work for the NHS in England on oral health assessment in clinical practice underlined the need for a comprehensive and evidence-based approach [15] and led to the development of an outline dental care pathway [16].

This work and subsequent development with the NHS in Scotland has shown that the caries side of a patient's treatment need must be carefully integrated with other oral health needs. A Scottish Dental Clinical Effectiveness Programme (SDCEP) Guideline Development Group has been examining these issues for some time and is at present consulting on draft guidance [17]. The key elements of the draft recommendations are that dentists should:

(1) conduct a comprehensive assessment of the individual for each patient, including (a) social history, dental history and medical history, and keep these records up to date, (b) assessment of each patient's experience of, and attitude to, dental care, (c) assessment of each patient's ability to understand the care provided;

(2) conduct a comprehensive clinical assessment of the oral health status for each patient including appropriate assessment of (a) caries and restorations using the ICDAS codes, and (b) appropriate radiographic assessments, the views taken being based on initial clinical findings;

(3) assign an overall risk level for each patient on the basis of assessment of the caries status, oral mucosa and periodontal tissues;

(4) assign a recall interval for each patient that is based on the individual's risk profile

(5) write a long-term personal care plan for each patient that is specific for the individual patient, containing advice for the patient and, if required, a summary of the preventive treatments, operative treatments and maintenance options planned.

The SDCEP group and team have also produced the risk assessment process overview (fig. 3) which demonstrates how the tooth-related caries information should be combined with a broader patient view to inform the choice of recall interval.

Developments in the USA

In the USA, 'Caries management by risk assessment (CAMBRA)' has represented a paradigm shift in the management of dental caries [18] and now represents a

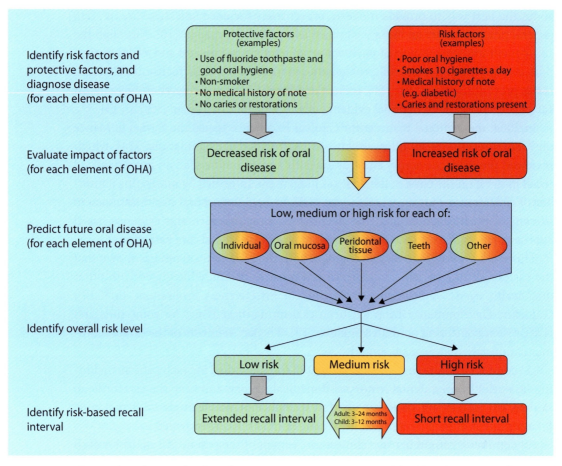

Fig. 3. Flow diagram for the risk assessment process across oral health informing recall interval selection. OHA = Oral health assessment.

personalized approach. It treats dental caries as an infectious disease that is curable and preventable. The science supporting CAMBRA has been present for quite some time [19]; however, its clinical adoption, until recently, remained slow. This group, particularly the Western CAMBRA coalition in the early stages has built a special collaboration of diverse groups of independent organizations based in their region of the USA. This coalition, which has formed an interorganizational collaborative, has evolved over the years and has led to significant progress in the clinical adoption of CAMBRA. This collaboration has spread across the USA to now include mid-US and Eastern CAMBRA groups. The preventive focus advocated by the group is professional, intense and patient centred. Some clarity is needed on the strength of evidence underlying some of the procedures advocated however as the level of evidence supporting some of the interventions used is, at present, weaker than the SDCEP grading system would recognize.

At the same time, a number of US dental schools have introduced a preventive caries management emphasis in their undergraduate courses and have developed caries risk assessment and preventive caries management forms for their student clinics. The speed of adoption has been limited in many schools, but the formation of a cariology special interest group within the American Association for Dental Education has now galvanized the pace of action.

ICDAS Committee Overview to Support Clinical Practice

The ICDAS framework for patient-centred caries management (fig. 2) is designed to allow the dentist and the dental team to integrate information from all the elements in order to synthesize this at both the lesion and the patient levels in order to plan care.

The detail of what information to collect for each framework element is outlined (as indicated above) in the respective chapters of this book. It is, however, useful to outline some of the way in which the terminology in this area is being used and to show how information collected from the clinical visual assessments can be combined with information from both lesion detection aids and care planning aids. This collation has been developed by the ICDAS Committee over several years, and a consensus was achieved at a meeting in Bogota, Colombia, at the end of 2008.

Lesion-Related Information at the Tooth Surface
In order to plan treatment, a clinician needs to be able to make a diagnosis at the lesion level. The chapter by Longbottom et al [this vol., pp. 209–216] sets out consensus definitions for many of the terms, but the key terms are restated here, as it is important to understand the differences between *lesion detection, lesion assessment* and *diagnosis*.

- *Caries/carious lesion:* a caries /carious lesion is a detectable change in the tooth structure that results from the biofilm-tooth interactions occurring due to the disease caries
- *Lesion detection:* a process involving the recognition (and/or recording), traditionally by optical or physical means, of changes in enamel and/or dentine and/or cementum, which are consistent with having been caused by the caries process
- *Lesion assessment:* the evaluation of the characteristics of a caries lesion, once it has been detected; these characteristics may include optical, physical, chemical or biochemical parameters, such as colour, size or surface integrity
- *Caries diagnosis:* the human professional summation of all the signs and symptoms of disease to arrive at an identification of the past or present occurrence of the disease caries

So *lesion diagnosis* is the process by which the clinician, acting with human professional judgement, sums all the signs and symptoms of caries relating to a particular tooth surface – whether it be derived from visual detection of the lesion, additional

Sites of caries (1–4)	Stages of caries (0–3)			
	0 **No disease** ICDAS definition 0	1 **Initial** lesion ICDAS definitions 1 + 2	2 **Moderate** lesion ICDAS definitions 3 + 4	3 **Extensive** lesion ICDAS definition 5 + 6
1 Pit and fissure surfaces	1.0	1.1	1.2	1.3
2 Approximal surfaces	2.0	2.1	2.2	2.3
3 Cervical + smooth surfaces	3.0	3.1	3.2	3.3
4 Root surfaces	4.0	4.1	4.2	4.3

Fig. 4. Simplified format of ICDAS codes as part of a caries classification system for general practice and IT-based record systems (following an American Dental Association workshop in 2008).

information from radiography (or some other detection aid) or from one-time activity assessment, to arrive at a clear picture of both the extent and nature of caries in one part of a tooth.

The information to support diagnosis is recorded using appropriate scoring codes (such as the ICDAS codes). The format does not need to be too complicated and, for general practice use, a simplified table, grouping together ICDAS codes into 3 colour-coded stages of caries has been developed (fig. 4). This builds on the consensus development work brokered by the American Dental Association. The addition of colour coding is seen as helpful for communications with patients from the dental team.

Lesion prognosis is a further important consideration in treatment planning. Once again a clear understanding of the terminology is useful here, particularly *lesion activity* and *lesion prognosis*.

- *Lesion activity (net progression):* the summation of the dynamics of the caries process resulting in the net loss, over time, of mineral from a caries lesion – i.e. there is active lesion progression (the clinical reality here is of a lesion in a state of disease progression, as opposed to disease regression)
- *An active lesion:* a caries lesion from which, over a specified period of time, there is net mineral loss, i.e. the lesion is progressing (in this case, an active lesion refers to a one-point-in-time characterization of the lesion, using particular lesion parameters as indicative of lesion progression)
- *Lesion prognosis:* the likely future behaviour of (or clinical outcome for) a specific caries lesion, over a specified time period, as assessed by a clinician – taking into

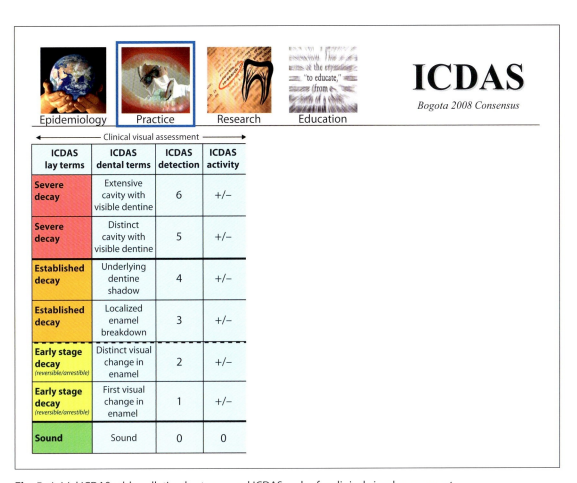

Fig. 5. Initial ICDAS table collating lay terms and ICDAS codes for clinical visual assessment.

account the summation of the multiple factors impacting on the (future) possible progression, arrest or regression of the lesion (some of the information needed to make these assessments is outlined in the chapters on patient caries risk assessment, dentition and lesion history) and patient behavioural assessment, as there is a need here to synthesize some of the material collected at the tooth level with factors identified at the patient level; the 2-way arrow in the central part of figure 2 between lesion prognosis and prognosis for patient indicates the need to link lesion-level and patient-level information.

The initial ICDAS table outlined in figure 5 collates standardized lay terms for dental decay with codes for clinical visual assessment – that is both ICDAS detection codes and ICDAS activity status. (The table is focussed upon the clinical practice use of ICDAS, hence the emphasis 'box' at the top of fig. 5.)

As has been stated previously and outlined in the chapters on lesion detection aids, some lesions cannot be detected by clinical examination alone, even when a skilled

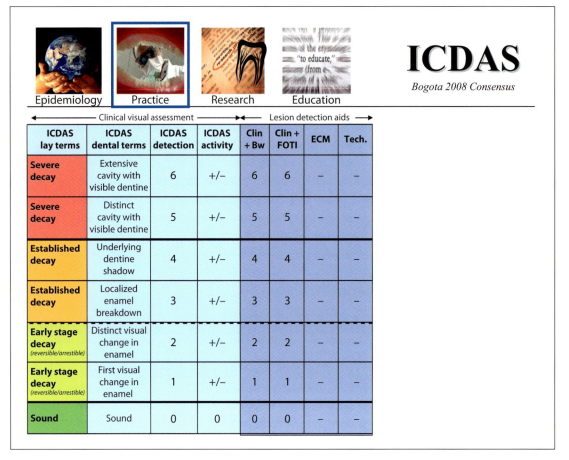

Fig. 6. Intermediate ICDAS table: clinical visual assessment and lesion detection aids. Clin. = Clinical; BW = bitewing; FOTI = fibre-optic transillumination; ECM = electronic caries monitor; tech. = technological.

examiner has unlimited time looking at a dry, clean field. For this reason, in planning treatment there is a need to carefully build on the information derived from clinical visual assessment by adding additional, complementary information derived from the increasing range of lesion detection aids available.

The intermediate ICDAS table outlined in figure 6 adds information from lesion detection aids to the existing clinical visual assessment data. Note that there are cells provided for radiographic information, fibre-optic transillumination information as well as electronic caries monitors and any other, future, technologies with diagnostic utility.

Patient-Related Information
Moving now away from the necessary detail on individual lesions on specific surfaces of particular teeth, it is important to also consider the wider patient perspective. The

detail about what patient level information is needed to inform personalized treatment planning is outlined in the chapters on patient caries risk assessment, dentition and lesion history and patient behavioural assessment. This information should be recorded appropriately in the patient records and be synthesized firstly to build an overall patient assessment and prognosis and secondly in order to link with the lesion level assessments in order to construct the item-by-item plan most appropriate to this patient at this time. The behavioural factors are frequently ignored, but it is these that will determine what part the patient is likely to play in changing and maintaining the health behaviours that will be critical to long-term caries control.

The *prognosis for the patient* is essentially derived from all the background information collected from dental, medical and social histories and is a *prediction of the probable course and outcome of the disease.*

Integrated, Personalized Treatment Planning
The treatment plan is constructed as a prioritized, personalized list of types of care and individual procedures. Although many have indicated how attractive automated decision tools might be in this area, with software following automated rules for preventive and restorative treatments and recall intervals, the evidence that we have to date is not yet sufficiently precise to allow such automated calculations. The guidance on recall intervals from the National Institute for Clinical Excellence [14] warns us specifically that when synthesizing information across dental caries and then across periodontal and oral medicine risks, we still need to employ the clinical judgement of a dentist.

The full ICDAS table, outlined in figure 7, adds information derived from care planning aids to the previously recorded information from clinical visual assessment and from lesion detection aids.

Figure 7 provides for entry of a patient's caries risk status (assessed as high, medium or low), the entry of results from any technological method(s) of assessing caries activity, as well as whether the care range is likely to involve preventive treatment options, operative treatment options or both. The final cells allow for the recording of monitoring lesions over time (ICDAS monitor – lesions may be p = progressing, a = arrested or r = regressing). This does not dictate the specific format for data entry for all tooth surfaces, it rather presents the core information that should be recorded and collated to inform personalized treatment planning.

Once again, it is important to have a clear understanding of the definitions of the key terms in this area.
- *Lesion behaviour:* defined in terms of what changes, if any, occur in the status of a lesion over time in response to the balance between demineralization and remineralization [a lesion can, between 2 time points: (a) progress (exhibit net mineral loss), (b) arrest, i.e. remain unchanged (static/stable) or (c) regress (exhibit net mineral gain); at a further (third and/or subsequent) time point, the lesion can exhibit any of the above 3 changes, and hence (d) undergo oscillations in status]

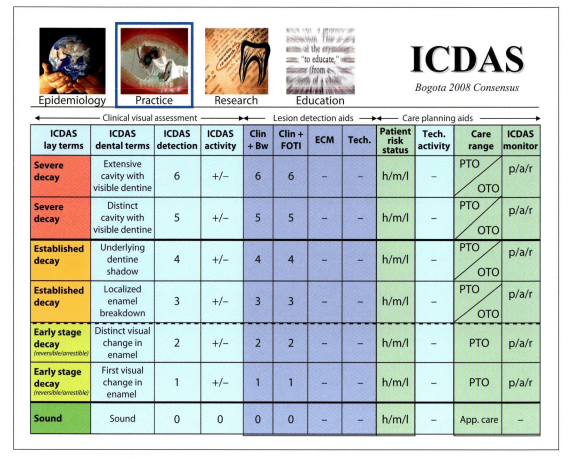

Fig. 7. Full ICDAS table: clinical visual assessment, lesion detection aids and care planning aids. h = High; m = medium; l = low; PTO = preventive treatment option; OTO = operative treatment option; p = progressing; a = arrested; r = regressing; for explanation of other abbreviations, see legend of figure 6.

- *Monitoring of a caries/carious lesion:* the assessment, over time, of one or more of the characteristics of a caries lesion to assess if any changes have occurred in that lesion
- *An active lesion:* a caries lesion, from which, over a specified period of time, there is net mineral loss, i.e. the lesion is progressing (this use of the term here relates to assessment at 2 or more time points, of specific lesion parameters/characteristics, when monitoring a lesion)
- *An arrested or inactive lesion:* a lesion which is not undergoing net mineral loss – i.e. the caries process in a specific lesion is no longer progressing (this may be assessed, by comparison/monitoring of lesion characteristics over a specified time period, as being consistent with those of lesion arrest)

- *Lesion regression:* the net gain of calcified material to the structure of a caries lesion, replacing that which was previously lost through caries demineralization
- *Remineralized caries lesion:* a caries lesion which exhibits evidence of having undergone net mineral gain – i.e. there is replacement of mineral which was previously lost due to the caries process

Treatment planning options can now be selected on the basis of comprehensive information about this patient at this specific time point and taking into account their caries history and the likely prognosis. The options are set out in the following sections (covering specific options): 'Background level care', 'Traditional preventive treatment options', 'Novel preventive treatment options', 'Traditional operative treatment options' and 'Novel operative treatment options'. Lastly, there is the chapter covering recall, reassessment and monitoring.

The philosophy employed in selecting options should be that which provides truly minimally invasive dentistry over the long term. Minimally invasive dentistry is supported by the emerging evidence and by international consensus; it has an international focus, from for example the Fédération Dentaire Internationale and others, and continues to be built on. This is a vitally important term, but one which means different things to different people in dentistry. Its definition should therefore be made very clear.

The minimally invasive dentistry approach stresses a preventive philosophy, individualized risk assessments, accurate, early detection of lesions, efforts to remineralize non-cavitated lesions with the prompt provision of preventive care in order to minimize operative intervention. When operative intervention is unequivocally required, typically for an active cavitated lesion, the procedure used should be as minimally invasive as possible.

What is not supported by the evidence, or international consensus, but which is sometimes *mislabelled* as *minimally invasive* is clinical activity in which small, early and inactive/arrested lesions are sought out and prematurely or unnecessarily subjected to operative intervention.

Research Issues in Personalized Treatment Planning

These include:
- integrating lesion detection and activity information with patient level caries risk estimates;
- further studies assessing the reliability of assessing caries risk factors in dental primary care across all age groups;
- the level of compliance of patients with recommended preventive procedures and behaviours, as well as with recall intervals;
- comparative, long-term, health-economic evaluation of the full range of treatment options.

Implementation Issues

Implementing research findings into general practice is a complex jigsaw puzzle which always presents both challenges and opportunities [20]. Issues around implementing the broad range of subjects covered by this book are covered in the chapter by Pitts [this vol., pp. 199–208]. The specific issues around personalized treatment planning include:

- skills around integrating and synthesizing information in a team setting;
- charting in more detail using a consistent system (for both dentists and nurses);
- appropriate development of dental practice IT systems and software;
- the prevailing restorative-dominated dental 'culture' in many places;
- declining cariology expertise available in dental education in many countries;
- payment/remuneration/compensation systems which do not incentivize preventive practice [21].

References

1 Pitts NB: 'ICDAS' – an international system for caries detection and assessment being developed to facilitate caries epidemiology, research and appropriate clinical management (editorial). Community Dental Health 2004;21:193–198.
2 Bader J, Shugars D: Understanding dentists' restorative treatment decisions. J Publ Health Dent 1992;52:102–110.
3 Elderton RJ: Clinical studies concerning re-restoration of teeth. Adv Dent Res 1990;4:4–9.
4 Evans RW, Pakdaman A, Dennison PJ, Howe ELC: The Caries Management System: an evidence-based preventive strategy for dental practitioners – application for adults. Aust Dent J 2008;53:83–92.
5 Tyas MJ, Anusavice KJ, Frencken JE, Mount GJ: Minimal intervention dentistry – a review. FDI commission project 1-97. Int Dent J 2000;50:1–12.
6 Bourgeois DM, Llodra JC, Nordblad A, Pitts NB: Report of the EGOHID I Project – selecting a coherent set of indicators for monitoring and evaluating oral health in Europe: criteria, methods and results from the EGOHID I Project. Community Dent Health 2008;25:4–11.
7 Bourgeois DM, Christensen LB, Ottolenghi L, Llodra JC, Pitts NB, Senakola E (eds): Health Surveillance in Europe – European Global Oral Health Indicators Development Project Oral Health Interviews and Clinical Surveys: Guidelines. Lyon, Lyon I University Press, 2008.
8 Pitts NB: Are we ready to move from operative to non-operative/preventive treatment of dental caries in clinical practice? Caries Res 2004;38:294–304.
9 Pendlebury M, Pitts NB, Clarkson JEC (eds): Clinical Examination and Record Keeping. London, Faculty of General Dental Practitioners, 2001.
10 Pitts NB: NHS dentistry: options for change in context: a personal overview of landmark document and what it could mean for the future of dental services. Br Dent J 2003;195:631–635.
11 Department of Health: Delivering better oral health: an evidence-based toolkit for prevention. London, Department of Health and British Association for the Study of Community Dentistry, 2007.
12 SIGN guideline No 47: Scottish Intercollegiate Guideline Network – preventing dental caries in children at high caries risk: targeted prevention of dental caries in the permanent teeth of 6–16 year olds presenting for dental care. December 2000. www.sign.ac.uk.
13 SIGN guideline No 83: Scottish Intercollegiate Guideline Network – prevention and management of dental decay in the pre-school child: a national clinical guideline. November 2005. www.sign.ac.uk.
14 National Collaborating Centre for Acute Care, National Institute for Clinical Excellence: Dental recall – recall interval between routine dental examinations: methods, evidence and guidance. London, Royal College of Surgeons of England, October 2004. www.nice.org.uk/CG019fullguideline.
15 Pitts NB: Oral health assessment in clinical practice: new perspectives on the need for a comprehensive and evidence based approach. Br Dent J 2005;198:317.

16 Hally JD, Pitts NB: Developing the first dental care pathway: the oral health assessment. Primary Dent Care 2006;12:117–121.
17 Scottish Dental Clinical Effectiveness Programme (SDCEP) draft guidance on comprehensive oral health assessment. 2009. http://www.sdcep.org.uk/index.aspx?o = 2336/.
18 Young DA, Buchanan PM, Lubman RG, Badway NN: New directions in interorganizational collaboration in dentistry: the CAMBRA coalition model. J Dent Educ 2007;71:595–600.
19 Young DA, Featherstone JB, Roth JR: Caries Management by Risk Assessment – a practitioner's guide. CDA J 2007;35:679–680.
20 Pitts NB: Understanding the jigsaw of evidence based dentistry. 3. Implementation of research findings. Evidence Based Dentistry 2004;5:60–64.
21 Diagnosis and management of dental caries throughout life. National Institutes of Health consensus development conference statement, March 26–28, 2001. J Dent Educ 2001;65:935–1184.

N.B. Pitts
Dental Health Services and Research Unit, University of Dundee
Mackenzie Building, Kirsty Semple Way
Dundee DD2 4BF (UK)
Tel. +44 1382 420067, Fax +44 382 420051, E-Mail n.b.pitts@cpse.dundee.ac.uk

Background Level Care

N.B. Pitts

Dental Health Services and Research Unit, University of Dundee, Dundee, UK

Abstract

The framework enabled by the International Caries Detection and Assessment System to allow appropriate, patient-centred caries management includes a frequently encountered scenario in which a comprehensive assessment of the teeth and the patient reveals no lesions in need of active preventive or operative care. The issue addressed here is: what background care is appropriate for patients attending a dental practice for routine caries care who, at present, appear to have no active or progressing caries lesions? It is proposed that, in addition to the use of criteria for lesion extent, treatment planning systems should also express the results of lesion assessments in terms of background level care (BLC), preventive treatment options and operative treatment options. The specific treatment options recommended for specific lesions and patients will depend upon a variety of other factors, including lesion activity, monitoring lesion behaviour over time and a range of other prognostic factors. Over recent decades, there has been comparatively little focus on appropriate BLC in a general practice setting. There are a range of issues around the need to support caries prevention and health maintenance from a behavioural and patient-focussed perspective. Even if a patient is deemed to be at low risk of future caries at a particular examination, there is a need for maintenance care. Intrinsic issues which need to be managed for both patients and their caries lesions in this patient group are: (1) the possibility of a change in caries risk status and (2) the impact of incorrect lesion assessments/diagnoses.

Copyright © 2009 S. Karger AG, Basel

The framework enabled by the International Caries Detection and Assessment System (ICDAS) to allow appropriate, patient-centred caries management – based on the application of best current evidence and practice – which is outlined in the chapter by Pitts and Richards [this vol., pp. 128–143] includes a frequently encountered scenario in which a comprehensive assessment of the teeth and the patient reveals no lesions which are apparently in need of active preventive or operative care. The issue addressed in this chapter is: what background care is appropriate for people attending a dental practice for routine caries care who, at present, appear to have no active or progressing caries lesions?

A review of categorizing caries by the management option some 14 years ago [1] identified a range of systems and classifications used by clinicians (as well as epidemiologists and clinical research workers) to subdivide carious lesions into different grades. These systems were based on the depth of the lesion and/or the presence/absence of macroscopic cavitation. In order to improve upon the meaningfulness and comparability of such systems (in the light of increasing knowledge about the disease process, lesion behaviour and caries management options), the authors then proposed an iceberg metaphor for caries detection and a new system of categorization that differentiates between lesions which normally require operative intervention and those which do not. They proposed that, *in addition* to the use of any conventional criteria for lesion extent, diagnostic and treatment planning systems should also allow the results of lesion assessments to be expressed in terms of (1) lesions for which appropriate non-invasive *preventive care is advised* and (2) lesions for which *operative care is advised*.

Over the intervening years, this nomenclature has been in use in a number of countries, while in Scandinavia a similar 'non-operative care/operative care' dichotomy has also been used extensively. With further international harmonization through the work of the ICDAS Committee [2], in a treatment planning context, these two types of clinical management option are increasingly now referred to as *preventive treatment options* and *operative treatment options* – for details see the chapters by Longbottom et al. [this vol., pp. 149–155 and 156–163] and Ricketts and Pitts [this vol., pp. 164–173 and 174–187].

A further review of the impact on planning appropriate care of 'diagnostic tools and measurements' some 12 years ago [3] represented the iceberg metaphor for understanding caries detected at different diagnostic thresholds and also determining the differing management options appropriate for the care of different types of active and inactive lesions. In this system, for patients with no obvious caries or no active lesions, *no active care* was advised. As this term has, in some quarters, stimulated debates about giving the impression of a dental practice failing to look after regularly attending patients by providing preventive maintenance care, it has been superseded by the term 'background level care' (BLC).

Current Caries Classification by Management Option

Figure 1 shows the way in which the iceberg metaphor is now presented with ICDAS caries detection codes on the front face of the caries 'cube' of modern caries measurement [4] providing the stages of lesion extent that can be generally subdivided into BLC, preventive treatment options and operative treatment options. The specific treatment options recommended for specific lesions in specific patients will depend upon a variety of other factors, including assessing lesion activity, monitoring lesion behaviour over time (fig. 1) and a range of other prognostic and patient-related factors [for further details, see the chapter by Pitts and Richards, this vol., pp. 128–143].

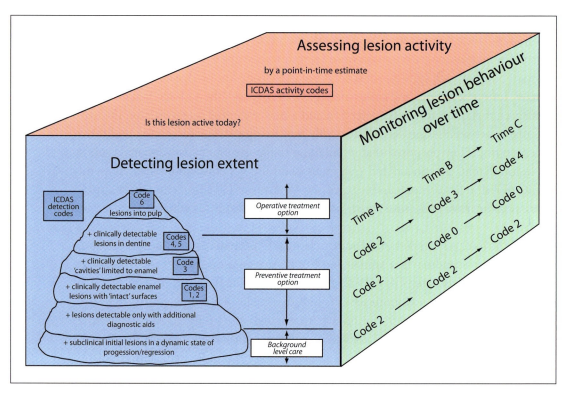

Fig. 1. The caries cube: relating the detection of lesion extent, assessment of lesion activity and monitoring of lesion behaviour over time.

Background Level Care

Over recent decades there has been comparatively little focus on specifying appropriate BLC in a general practice setting. While there is a short-term health economic temptation to simply say that 'no treatment is needed' and therefore patients do not need to be seen, there are also a range of issues around the need to support caries prevention and health maintenance from a behavioural and patient-focussed perspective. Even if a patient is deemed to be at low risk of future caries at a particular examination, there is a need for maintenance care. This is well documented in the treatment of periodontal disease with specific hygiene and maintenance phases of treatment. However, in clinical caries care this approach is less well described and evaluated. Secondary prevention and treatment of dental caries should focus on the management of the caries process over extended time periods for individual patients, with a minimally invasive, tissue-preserving approach [5].

The caries status of an individual patient has to be assessed in a holistic sense in parallel with the current risk status for both periodontal disease and oral mucosal lesions, particularly when assessing recall intervals [6]. The other intrinsic issues which need to be managed for both patients and their caries lesions in this group are (1) the possibility of a change in caries risk status and (2) the impact of incorrect lesion assessments/diagnoses. These issues should be seen in the context of a continuing cycle of comprehensive oral health assessments for new patients, followed by serial *oral health reviews* in continuing care [6, 7].

The Possibility of a Change in Caries Risk Status

A minority of, but still some, patients who have been classified as having a low caries risk will inevitably develop new caries lesions over time. This may either be because of a misclassification of risk status [see the chapter by Twetman and Fontana, this vol., pp. 91–101] or because their risk category has genuinely changed over time. Changes in salivary flow as a consequence of new or changed medications are a classic example of this sometimes silent shift in risk status.

The Impact of Incorrect Lesion Assessments/Diagnoses

Some individual patients are very well controlled in terms of not developing either active lesions or new caries. In these cases, the dentist need not do anything above reinforcing general preventive advice in a personalized way, while maintaining vigilance for any changes in risk status. However, the clinical diagnosis of dental caries is a complex process, involving the steps of detection, assessment and frequently monitoring, and is not an exact science, even for the diligent practitioner. Inherent deficiencies with current lesion detection methods [see the chapters by Topping and Pitts, this vol., pp. 15–41, and Neuhaus et al., this vol., pp. 42–51 and 52–61] can impact upon planning the care of individuals by allowing false-negative diagnoses of hidden occlusal dentine lesions and approximal cavities on the one hand, whilst generating some false-positive diagnoses on sound surfaces leading to inappropriate decisions to restore on the other [3].

BLC should be relevant to the patient, the type of dental practice, the health system under which the practice operates as well as the setting and country in which care is delivered. Essentially BLC should provide maintenance and monitoring of preventive caries control between routine visits [see the chapter by Clarkson et al., this vol., pp. 188–198]. This care should be provided in the knowledge that there is a possibility that a patient's caries risk status may change and that some lesion assessments and diagnoses may be incorrect.

Research and Implementation Considerations

The adoption of the *additional* nomenclature of BLC (as well as preventive and operative treatment options), over and above lesion detection and activity codes, together with this approach to planning personalized caries care, should aid communications between the different groups of staff involved in caries detection, assessment, diagnosis and monitoring within the clinical practice domain. The system will also assist communication between patient and dental team and links from practice to research, education and public health.

BLC supports long-term, personalized caries prevention and health maintenance from a behavioural, risk management and patient-focussed perspective.

References

1 Pitts NB, Longbottom C: Preventive care advised (PCA)/operative care advised (OCA) – categorising caries by the management option. Community Dent Oral Epidemiol 1995;23:55–59.
2 ICDAS – International Caries Detection and Assessment System. www.icdas.org.
3 Pitts NB: Diagnostic tools and measurements – impact on appropriate care. Community Dent Oral Epidemiol 1997;25:24–35.
4 Pitts NB: Modern concepts of caries measurement. J Dent Res 2004;83(spec iss C):43–47.
5 Selwitz RH, Ismail AI, Pitts NB: Dental caries. Lancet 2007;369:51–59.
6 National Collaborating Centre for Acute Care, National Institute for Clinical Excellence (NICE): Dental recall – recall interval between routine dental examinations: methods, evidence and guidance. Royal College of Surgeons of England, London, October 2004. www.nice.org.uk/CG019fullguideline.
7 Hally JD, Pitts NB: Developing the first dental care pathway: the oral health assessment. Primary Dent Care 2006;12:117–121.

N.B. Pitts
Dental Health Services and Research Unit, University of Dundee
Mackenzie Building, Kirsty Semple Way
Dundee DD2 4BF (UK)
Tel. +44 1382 420067, Fax +44 1382 420051, E-Mail n.b.pitts@cpse.dundee.ac.uk

Traditional Preventive Treatment Options

C. Longbottom[a] · K. Ekstrand[b] · D. Zero[c]

[a]Dental Health Services and Research Unit, University of Dundee, UK; [b]University of Copenhagen, Copenhagen, Denmark; [c]Indiana University School of Dentistry, Indianapolis, Ind., USA

Abstract

Preventive treatment options can be divided into primary, secondary and tertiary prevention techniques, which can involve patient- or professionally applied methods. These include: oral hygiene (instruction), pit and fissure sealants ('temporary' or 'permanent'), fluoride applications (patient- or professionally applied), dietary assessment and advice (modification), other measures to help remineralize demineralized tissue and other measures to help modify the biofilm to reduce the cariogenic challenge. There is a considerable body of strong evidence supporting the use of specific techniques for primary prevention of caries in children, e.g. pit and fissure sealants and topically applied fluorides (including patient-applied fluoride toothpastes and professionally applied fluoride varnishes), but limited strong evidence for these techniques for secondary prevention – i.e. where early to established lesions with ICDAS codes 1–4 (and also the severer lesions coded 5 or 6) are involved – and in relation to adults. This lack of evidence reflects a shortage of high-quality trials in the area, as opposed to a series of good studies showing no effect. Since there is also limited longitudinal evidence supporting conventional operative care, and since controlling the caries process *prior* to first restoration is the key to breaking the repair cycle and improving care for patients, future research should address the shortcomings in the current level of supporting evidence for the various traditional preventive treatment options.

Copyright © 2009 S. Karger AG, Basel

This chapter sets out to provide an overview of the various preventive treatment options available to the clinician and help frame the choices for different age groups and the current strength of published evidence supporting these interventions. The grading recommended by the Scottish Clinical Effectiveness Programme is employed [for further details, see the chapter by Pitts, this vol., pp. 1–14].

'Preventive treatments' can be differentiated into three classical, sometimes overlapping, categories: primary prevention, secondary prevention and tertiary prevention. Primary prevention includes those measures which prevent the development of the clinical signs of caries in the absence of disease, i.e. prevent the initiation of the disease. Secondary prevention centres on the prompt and efficacious treatment of disease at an early stage and includes measures which arrest and/or reverse the

Table 1. ICDAS lesion detection codes: 0- to 6-year-olds (primary dentition)

Prevention	0 (sound) with caries risk: low/moderate/high	1 + 2 (initial lesion)	3 + 4 (moderate lesion)	5 + 6 (extensive lesion)
Primary (grade 1)	background/ background + / background ++	background	background	background
Secondary (grade 2)	–	F prof. applied (R_w); pit and fissure sealants (R_w); enhanced OHI (R_e)	for surfaces accessible to cleaning of lesion surface: F prof. applied (R_e); enhanced OHI (R_e)	for surfaces accessible to cleaning of lesion surface: F prof. applied (R_e); enhanced OHI (R_e)
Hybrid (grades 2 + 3)	–	–	–	ART (R_w)

The strength of the evidence for a particular preventive therapy will vary according to which stage of caries is being addressed. OHI = Oral hygiene instruction; atraumatic restorative treatment (ART) is seen as traditional in some countries and novel in others.

caries process after initiation of clinical signs. Tertiary prevention involves measures which remove irreversibly damaged tooth tissue and replace it in such a way as to prevent further progress of the caries process. Some secondary and tertiary preventive options involve a 'hybrid' interaction of non-operative and operative procedures.

There are several general categories of preventive treatment options which are seen by many in the profession as 'traditional'. These may be patient applied or professionally applied and are:
1 oral hygiene (instruction);
2 pit and fissure sealants (considered as 'temporary' or 'permanent');
3 fluoride applications (patient or professionally applied);
4 dietary assessment and advice (modification);
5 other measures to help remineralize demineralized tissue;
6 other measures to help modify the biofilm to reduce the cariogenic challenge.

Tables 1–4 and the appendix provide a summary (guidance) of the preventive treatment options available for the different stages of caries lesions – as designated by the International Caries Detection and Assessment System (ICDAS) criteria – and the summarized level of evidence for each of the 3 categories of caries-preventive treatments following a review of the key systematic reviews and guidance documents in the literature [1–17].

Table 2. ICDAS lesion detection codes: 6- to 12-year-olds (permanent dentition)

Prevention	0 (sound) with caries risk: low/moderate/high	1 + 2 (initial lesion)	3 + 4 (moderate lesion)	5 + 6 extensive lesion)
Primary (grade 1)	background/ background +/ background ++; 'background' includes 'lateral' brushing of erupting 1st and 2nd molar teeth	background	background	background
Secondary (grade 2)	–	F prof. applied (R_w); pit and fissure sealants (R_w); enhanced OHI (R_w), especially for erupting molar teeth	pit and fissure sealants (R_w)	–
Hybrid (grades 2 + 3)	–	–	sealant restoration (R_e)	sealant restoration (R_e)

For the primary dentition in 6- to 12-year-olds, see table 1. OHI = Oral hygiene instruction. In addition to the background, background + and background ++ preventive treatment options (above), the following options can be used/recommended for all patients above 6 years old where the clinician judges it appropriate to the caries risk of the patient: xylitol as a non-sugar sweetener in the diet (R_w); sugar-free chewing gum and polyol-containing chewing gum (R_w); sugar-free medicines (R_w); chlorhexidine varnish (R_w); sucking of fluoride tablets (R_e).

Tables 1–4 address 4 age group bands, which reflect the developing (primary and mixed) child dentition, as well as the maturing and mature adult dentition. The 'borders' of these age group bands are not meant to be definitive but are approximate and can vary between individual patients as biological and chronological ages may not be perfectly matched.

For tables 1–4, the following applies regarding preventive treatment options:
- background level = parent and patient dental health education (R_s), plus oral hygiene instruction (R_s; when including the use of fluoride dentifrice with locally appropriate concentration), plus generalized dietary assessment and motivation (R_e; compatible with prevention using a common risk factor approach);
- background + level = background (above) plus professionally applied fluoride (R_s), plus enhanced oral hygiene instruction (including flossing where appropriate; R_s), plus enhanced patient-specific dietary assessment and motivation (R_w);
- background ++ level = background + (above) plus pit and fissure sealants (R_s).

Table 3. ICDAS lesion detection codes: 12- to 20-year-olds

Prevention	0 (sound) with caries risk: low/moderate/high	1 + 2 (initial lesion)	3 + 4 (moderate lesion)	5 + 6 (extensive lesion)
Primary (grade 1)	background/ background +/ background ++; 'background' includes 'lateral' brushing of erupting 2nd molar teeth	background	background	background
Secondary (grade 2)	–	F prof. applied (R_w); pit and fissure sealants (R_w); enhanced OHI (R_w), especially for erupting 2nd molar teeth	pit and fissure sealants (R_w)	–
Hybrid (grades 2 + 3)	–	–	sealant restoration (R_e)	sealant restoration (R_e)

OHI = Oral hygiene instruction.

Within the tables, recommendations are based on reviews of the evidence according to the Scottish Clinical Effectiveness Programme classification with:

R_s = recommendations supported by strong evidence with limited bias;
R_w = recommendations supported by weak evidence with some potential for bias;
R_e = recommendations based on a consensus of expert opinion.

It should be borne in mind, for comparative purposes, that using rigorous systematic review methodology and robust grading, the evidence supporting conventional operative caries management is limited and there is a wealth of evidence about the limited durability of conventional restorative care [18]. Controlling the caries process prior to the first restoration of teeth is the key to breaking the repair cycle and improving care for patients (fig. 1).

Conclusion

Tables 1–4 provide the appropriate available preventive treatment options for each of the ICDAS lesion severity codes (and erupting teeth) for each of the 3 prevention

Table 4. ICDAS lesion detection codes: ≥20-year-olds

Prevention	0 (sound) with caries risk: low/moderate/high	1 + 2 (initial lesion)	3 + 4 (moderate lesion)	5 + 6 (extensive lesion)
Primary (grade 1)	background/ background +/ background ++; 'background' includes 'lateral' brushing of erupting 3rd molar teeth	background	background	background
Secondary (grade 2)	–	F prof. applied (R_e); pit and fissure sealants (R_e); enhanced OHI (R_e)	pit and fissure sealants (R_e); enhanced OHI (R_e)	for root caries: F prof. applied (R_e); enhanced OHI (R_e)
Hybrid (grades 2 + 3)	–	–	sealant restoration (R_e)	for coronal caries: sealant restoration (R_e)

OHI = Oral hygiene instruction.

categories. The appendix gives a list of traditional preventive treatment options. The clinician should decide, using all the other information about the caries risk of the patient and other relevant information, which particular option is most appropriate for a given lesion in a given patient.

Further Research

The following are suggested as possible areas for further research, using robust methodological designs, into the traditional preventive treatment options:

1 the use of non-professional and professional interdental cleaning for the primary and secondary prevention of approximal caries in primary and permanent dentitions;
2 the use of pit and fissure sealants in primary teeth, including ICDAS detection code 3, 4 and 5 lesions;
3 the use of all traditional preventive treatment options, individually, in adults (ages ≥20 years);
4 the use of combinations of preventive treatment options in children and adults.

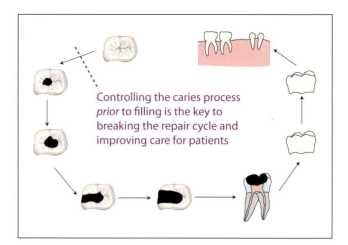

Fig. 1. The restorative cycle/spiral.

Implementation Priorities

Barriers to implementation of preventive treatment options include:
1   the traditional restoration-only culture embedded in many parts of dentistry;
2   the lack of incentives within many dental remuneration systems.

These barriers may be overcome by concerted professional activity, by the continuing development of consensus guidelines informed by the evolving evidence and by a greater use of a range of health professionals within and outside dentistry to deliver effective interventions.

Appendix

The following specific procedures are currently available in each traditional preventive treatment option category:

oral hygiene instruction: toothbrushing; specific 'lateral' toothbrushing of erupting molar teeth; flossing; other interdental cleaning aids;

pit and fissure sealants: resin-based systems; cement-based (temporary) sealants;

fluoride applications – patient-applied: dentifrice (various F ppm and types of F); mouthrinse;

fluoride applications – professionally applied: varnishes; gels; solutions;

dietary assessment and advice: verbal assessment and advice; written data collection (diet diary); written advice;

other remineralizing agents: sugar-free chewing gum; polyol gums;

other antimicrobial agents: chlorhexidine;

'hybrid' preventive/operative options: sealant restorations (preventive resin restorations).

References

1 Ahovuo-Saloranta A, Hiiri A, Nordblad A, Mäkelä M, Worthington HV: Pit and fissure sealants for preventing dental decay in the permanent teeth of children and adolescents. Cochrane Database Syst Rev 2008;4: CD001830. DOI: 10.1002/14651858.CD001830.pub3.

2 American Dental Association Council on Scientific Affairs: Professionally applied topical fluoride: evidence-based clinical recommendations. J Am Dent Assoc 2006;137:1151–1159.

3 American Dental Association Council on Scientific Affairs: Evidence-based clinical recommendations for the use of pit-and-fissure sealants. J Am Dent Assoc 2008;139:257–268.

4 Bader J, Shugars DA: The evidence supporting alternative management strategies for early occlusal caries and suspected dentinal caries. J Evid Based Dent Pract 2006;6:91–100.

5 Benson PE, Parkin N, Millett DT, Dyer F, Vine S, Shah A: Fluorides for the prevention of white spots on teeth during fixed brace treatment. Cochrane Database Syst Rev 2004;3:CD003809. DOI: 10.1002/14651858.CD003809.pub2.

6 Deshpande A, Jadad AR: The impact of polyol-containing chewing gums on dental caries: a systematic review of original randomized controlled trials and observational studies. J Am Dent Assoc 2008;139: 1602–1614.

7 Hiiri A, Ahovuo-Saloranta A, Nordblad A, Mäkelä M: Pit and fissure sealants versus fluoride varnishes for preventing dental decay in children and adolescents. Cochrane Database Syst Rev 2006;4:CD003067. DOI: 10.1002/14651858.CD003067.pub2.

8 Marinho VCC, Higgins JPT, Sheiham A, Logan S: Combinations of topical fluoride (toothpastes, mouthrinses, gels, varnishes) versus single topical fluoride for preventing dental caries in children and adolescents. Cochrane Database Syst Rev 2004;1: CD002781. DOI: 10.1002/14651858.CD002781.pub2.

9 Marinho VCC, Higgins JPT, Logan S, Sheiham A: Fluoride gels for preventing dental caries in children and adolescents. Cochrane Database Syst Rev 2002;1: CD002280. DOI: 10.1002/14651858.CD002280.

10 Marinho VCC, Higgins JPT, Logan S, Sheiham A: Fluoride mouthrinses for preventing dental caries in children and adolescents. Cochrane Database Syst Rev 2003;3:CD002284. DOI: 10.1002/14651858. CD002284.

11 Marinho VCC, Higgins JPT, Logan S, Sheiham A: Fluoride toothpastes for preventing dental caries in children and adolescents. Cochrane Database Syst Rev 2003; 1:CD002278. DOI: 10.1002/14651858. CD002278.

12 Marinho VCC, Higgins JPT, Logan S, Sheiham A: Fluoride varnishes for preventing dental caries in children and adolescents. Cochrane Database Syst Rev 2002;1:CD002279. DOI: 10.1002/14651858. CD002279.

13 Marinho VCC, Higgins JPT, Sheiham A, Logan S: One topical fluoride (toothpastes, or mouthrinses, or gels, or varnishes) versus another for preventing dental caries in children and adolescents. Cochrane Database Syst Rev 2004;1:CD002780. DOI: 10.1002/14651858.CD002780.pub2.

14 Marinho VCC, Higgins JPT, Logan S, Sheiham A: Topical fluoride (toothpastes, mouthrinses, gels or varnishes) for preventing dental caries in children and adolescents. Cochrane Database Syst Rev 2003; 4:CD002782. DOI: 10.1002/14651858.CD002782.

15 National Institutes of Health Consensus Development Conference Panel: National Institutes of Health consensus development conference statement: diagnosis and management of dental caries throughout life. J Dent Educ 2001;65:944–1179.

16 Scottish Intercollegiate Guideline Network: Preventing dental caries in children at high caries risk: targeted prevention of dental caries in the permanent teeth of 6–16 year olds presenting for dental care. SIGN guideline No 47. December 2000. www.sign.ac.uk.

17 Scottish Intercollegiate Guideline Network: Prevention and management of dental decay in the preschool child: a national clinical guideline. SIGN guideline No 83. November 2005. www.sign.ac.uk.

18 Elderton RJ: Clinical studies concerning rerestoration of teeth. Adv Dent Res 1990;4:4–9.

C. Longbottom
Dental Health Services and Research Unit, University of Dundee
Mackenzie Building, Kirsty Semple Way
Dundee DD2 4BF (UK)
Tel. +44 1382 420064, Fax +44 1382 420051, E-Mail c.longbottom@cpse.dundee.ac.uk

Novel Preventive Treatment Options

C. Longbottom[a] · K. Ekstrand[b] · D. Zero[c] · M. Kambara[d]

[a]Dental Health Services and Research Unit, University of Dundee, Dundee, UK; [b]University of Copenhagen, Copenhagen, Denmark; [c]Indiana University School of Dentistry, Indianapolis, Ind., USA; [d]Department of Preventive and Community Dentistry, Osaka Dental University, Osaka, Japan

Abstract

A number of novel preventive treatment options which, as with traditional methods, can be differentiated into 3 categories of prevention (primary, secondary and tertiary), have been and are being currently investigated. Those reviewed are either commercially available or appear relatively close to that point. These include: approximal sealants; fluoride applications, including slow-release devices; measures to help remineralize demineralized tissue, including 3 different methods of delivering amorphous calcium phosphate; measures to help modify the biofilm to reduce the cariogenic challenge, including ozone therapy and probiotics; measures to increase enamel resistance to demineralization, including laser treatment of enamel, and a novel 'hybrid' technique for the treatment of primary molar caries which involves 'overlapping' of secondary and tertiary prevention – the Hall technique. Although many of these techniques show considerable promise and dentists should be aware of these developments and follow their progress, the evidence for each of these novel preventive treatment options is currently insufficient to make widespread recommendations. Changes in dental practice should be explored to see how oral health can be best supported through novel preventive systems. Further research is also required involving double-blind randomized controlled trials in order to bring further benefits of more effective caries control to patients. Implementation in practice should follow promptly as new techniques are shown to be clinically valuable for individual patients.

Copyright © 2009 S. Karger AG, Basel

This chapter sets out to provide an overview of a number of novel preventive treatment options being developed in order to help clinicians better control the caries process in the future. Key published studies are identified and a novel approach to preventive practice in Japan is outlined. As with traditional preventive methods, the novel options which have been and are being currently investigated can be differentiated into the 3 fundamental categories of prevention (primary, secondary and tertiary). Primary prevention includes those measures which prevent the development of the clinical signs of caries in the absence of disease, i.e. prevent the initiation of the disease. Secondary prevention centres on the prompt and efficacious treatment of disease at an early stage and includes measures which arrest and/or reverse the caries process after initiation of clinical signs. Tertiary prevention involves measures which remove irreversibly damaged tooth tissue and replace it in such a way as to prevent further progression of the caries process. Some secondary and tertiary preventive options involve a 'hybrid' interaction of non-operative and operative procedures. The list of novel options below is not exhaustive but covers those techniques which are either commercially available or appear relatively close to that point.

These techniques fall within most of the general categories of preventive treatment options listed in the chapter by Longbottom et al. [this vol., pp. 149–155], with some minor modifications, and may be patient applied or professionally applied. They are:
1. approximal sealants;
2. fluoride applications;
3. measures to help remineralize demineralized tissue;
4. measures to help modify the biofilm to reduce the cariogenic challenge;
5. measures to increase enamel resistance to demineralization;
6. a novel 'hybrid' technique for the treatment of primary molar caries which involves 'overlapping' of secondary and tertiary prevention.

Approximal Sealants

This technique involves the use of temporary elective tooth separation to gain access to the approximal surface [1] prior to the application of an acid-etched retained sealant to seal a non-cavitated lesion, using a careful technique to avoid ledges at the sealant margins.

A number of in vitro studies have shown promising results, but, thus far, the only clinical studies which have been carried out have involved small numbers of patients, and there are insufficient data to make specific recommendations [2–4].

Fluoride Applications

Slow-Release Fluoride Devices

The use of slow-release fluoride devices for caries prevention has been suggested for some time. The technique involves the attachment (via acid-etched composite) of a small fluoride-containing device (e.g. a glass bead) to the crown of a tooth, generally to the buccal surface of an upper molar tooth, the device thereafter slowly releasing its fluoride over the period of a year or so into the intra-oral environment to maintain an elevated salivary fluoride concentration.

It is assumed that this elevated fluoride level in saliva helps to increase the plaque fluid fluoride concentration and thereby aids remineralization during sugar-mediated acid attacks on enamel.

Two recent reviews have concluded that, although the early results are promising, further randomized controlled trials are required before recommendations can be made [5, 6].

Measures to Help Remineralize Demineralized Tissue

Amorphous Calcium Phosphate

Until relatively recently the clinical use of calcium and phosphate ions to aid remineralization has not been successful mainly due to the low solubility of calcium phosphates, particularly in the presence of fluoride ions. However, 3 calcium-phosphate-based remineralization systems are now available commercially and have been the subject of a recent review [7].

Unstabilized amorphous calcium phosphate (Enamelon™) is used in the form of calcium ions and phosphate ions (sometimes in the presence of fluoride ions) applied separately so that amorphous calcium phosphate or calcium fluoride phosphate forms intra-orally. A number of studies have produced conflicting in vitro results in terms of the ability of this system to inhibit enamel demineralization or remineralize subsurface lesions. However, an in vivo study has demonstrated inhibition of root caries in a radiation therapy population, although there was no reduction in coronal caries relative to the control group [8]. A recent study on a similar population found that the system produced a significant benefit in preventing and remineralizing root caries [9].

A calcium sodium phosphosilicate bioactive glass – Novamin™ – is claimed to release calcium and phosphate ions intra-orally. However, Reynolds [7] could find no published studies showing an anticariogenic efficacy of the material, and none appear to have been published since.

The third material reviewed by Reynolds was casein-phosphopeptide-stabilized amorphous calcium phosphate – Recaldent™. Although the calcium, phosphate and fluoride ions are restabilized by the casein phosphopeptide from promoting calculus, they diffuse down concentration gradients into enamel subsurface lesions, thereby promoting remineralization. A considerable body of literature indicates that agents containing casein-phosphopeptide-stabilized amorphous calcium phosphate can help remineralize lesions in vitro, in situ and in vivo [7]. One randomized controlled clinical trial showed inhibition of caries progression and promotion of regression in approximal lesions in permanent teeth [10].

Hence, Reynolds [7] concluded that 'calcium phosphate remineralization technologies show promise as adjunctive treatments to fluoride therapy in the non-invasive management of early caries lesions'. However, a contemporaneous systematic review of the clinical efficacy of casein derivatives concluded that the clinical trial evidence was not yet sufficient to make conclusions regarding the long-term effectiveness of casein derivatives [11].

Measures to Help Modify the Biofilm to Reduce the Cariogenic Challenge

Ozone Therapy

The bactericidal properties of ozone are well known, and a device to apply ozone to carious lesions (across the International Caries Detection and Assessment System stages from 1 to 6) for coronal caries, as well as for root caries, is commercially available – Healozone.

However, two recent systematic reviews have both concluded that whilst laboratory studies have shown antimicrobial effects of ozone application, the in vivo studies have not achieved a strong level of efficacy, and, further, well-designed and -conducted double-blind clinical trials are required before a robust evaluation can be made of the use of ozone for the prevention and treatment of caries [12, 13] and recommendations can be given.

Probiotics

Probiotic bacteria are used to treat or prevent a broad range of human diseases, conditions and syndromes [14]. Their use in relation to caries relates to attempts at the replacement or displacement of cariogenic bacteria in the oral cavity [15].

A recent review of probiotics and oral health in children found that a number of studies indicated a 'hampering' effect on mutans streptococci and/or yeast [16]. In addition, the single study carried out in early childhood reported a significant caries reduction in 3- to 4-year-old children after 7 months of daily consumption of probiotic milk.

However, the authors concluded that further placebo-controlled trials that assess carefully selected and defined probiotic strains using standardized outcomes are needed before any clinical recommendations can be made. Similarly, a review by Meurman and Stamatova [17] concluded that hardly any randomized controlled trials had been conducted in this area and much more investigation was needed before any evidence-based conclusions can be drawn about whether probiotic therapy could be recommended for oral health purposes.

Measures to Increase Enamel Resistance to Demineralization

Laser Treatment of Enamel

Laboratory studies have shown that lasers can be used to modify the chemical composition of tooth enamel to render it less soluble and more resistant to demineralization [18–20].

However, there are no reports as yet of in vivo studies testing the efficacy of these lasers in preventing caries or reducing caries progression.

A Novel 'Hybrid' Technique for the Treatment of Primary Molar Caries Which Involves 'Overlapping' of Secondary and Tertiary Prevention

The Hall Technique

A general dental practitioner working in Scotland developed a novel method of placing preformed metal crowns (PMCs) on carious primary molar teeth using no local anaesthesia, no caries removal and no tooth preparation: the Hall technique. By completely covering the carious lesion and ensuring that the margins of the PMC were beneath the gingival crevice, the PMC effectively deprives the biofilm of nutrients and the caries process is halted (if pulpal infection has not already occurred or is so imminent as to be irreversible). Retrospective analysis of the practitioner's records indicated that survival rates for these PMCs were comparable to the values in the literature for the recognized conventional PMC placement technique used in the hands of specialist paediatric dentists [21].

A prospective randomized controlled trial was subsequently undertaken comparing the Hall technique with conventional restorations [22]. The results after 2 years demonstrated that Hall PMCs showed statistically significantly more favourable outcomes for pulpal health and restoration longevity than conventional restorations.

Further planned randomized controlled trials will enable evidence-based recommendations to be made regarding this novel approach to the secondary and tertiary prevention of International Caries Detection and Assessment System code 5 and 6 lesions in primary molar teeth.

Novel Approaches to Preventive Practice

Although many of the techniques outlined above show considerable promise and dentists should be aware of these developments and follow their progress, the evidence for each of these novel preventive treatment options is currently insufficient to make widespread recommendations. Further high-quality studies are being and will continue to be undertaken in order to develop better preventive treatment options. In the interim, changes in dental practice should be explored to see how oral health can be best supported by the use of novel preventive systems. Ideally, new methods should be evaluated in practice-based research networks and settings in addition to more conventional research and development pathways. Practice dynamics and patient communications should be arranged to facilitate a more preventive style of practice so as to be able to exploit current preventive treatment options and be ready to adopt those new techniques which are shown to have therapeutic and clinical benefit.

In Japan dental caries prevalence has decreased in recent years [23], and there is a perceived need to develop and evaluate new dental systems in clinics/practices which are linked to evidence from both epidemiological studies and dental science. In a country that has been used to high levels of caries, there is a need to establish models of practice which manage oral health for people with fewer, smaller lesions and maintains those without established dental caries in that state. If children have no occasion to visit dental clinics which are geared to provide only restorative care, there will be a declining awareness of dental health in the future. It follows that dentistry must change its focus [24, 25]. In the 20th century, dentistry was mostly concerned with the operative treatment of dental caries; however, in the 21st century dentistry must focus on maintaining unrestored teeth with caries controlled at the incipient disease level.

The philosophy promoting oral health is different from a traditional theory of prevention of oral diseases. For example lifestyle is important to oral health (eating and brushing habits for example), and patients should be encouraged towards positive health thinking. Oral health also needs social health which, for a given culture, means an optimal number of dentists, hygienists and dental offices, social security systems, and people motivated to maintain health.

Detection, Assessment and Control of Incipient Caries

We need to know the status of early carious changes before the disease becomes clinically obvious. If we could detect the subtle changes of a progressing incipient lesion in dental enamel, drilling would not be needed and we could utilize remineralization, which is potentially one of the most useful discoveries in dental science, as the preventive treatment option of choice. By using new technologies and estimation of caries activity, dentists should be able to select the optimal method of remineralization for their patients, for example, by changing the concentration and frequency of fluoride and other preventive materials. By utilizing this kind of up-to-date technology, dental treatment should become more evidence based, preventive and patient oriented.

An example of the sort of information that can inform preventive treatment choices is given in figure 1. Subjects at freshman grade (6 years old) in an elementary school in Osaka, Japan, receiving preventive care had the activity of incipient caries monitored using quantitative light-induced fluorescence over a period of 1.5 years. The activity (behaviour) of incipient caries (percentage of lesions assessed as active, arrested, recovering/regressing) in 3 subgroups, divided according to baseline caries scores, was found to be different. Recovery/regression showed the highest value (60.0%) in the high-health group, followed by the middle-health (35.0%) and then the low-health group (27.3%). On the other hand, the percentage of progressing lesions was highest in the low-health group (54.5%).

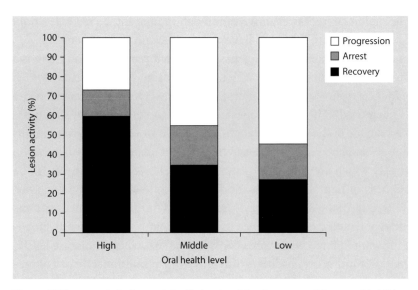

Fig. 1. Differences in lesion activity (behaviour) for 3 groups of 6-year-old children monitored over 1.5 years with quantitative light-induced fluorescence [Kambara et al., Osaka Dental University, unpubl. data].

Further Research

All of the promising novel techniques for preventive treatment listed above require further, carefully designed, randomized controlled trials to be carried out before evidence-based recommendations can be made in relation to their use.

Implementation Priorities

Implementation in practice should follow promptly once new techniques are shown to be clinically valuable for individual patients. Barriers to the utilization of new preventive approaches should be systematically overcome at both the dental practice and the health system levels.

References

1 Pitts NB, Longbottom C: Temporary elective tooth separation with special reference to the diagnosis and preventive management of equivocal approximal lesions. Quintessence Int 1987;18:563–573.
2 Gomez SS, Basili CP, Emilson CG: A 2-year clinical evaluation of sealed non-cavitated approximal posterior carious lesions in adolescents. Clin Oral Invest 2005;9:239–243.
3 Martignon S, Ekstrand KR, Ellwood R: Efficacy of sealing proximal early active lesions: an 18-month clinical study evaluated by conventional and subtraction radiography. Caries Res 2006;40:382–388.
4 Alkilzy M, Berndt C, Spleith CH: Therapeutic sealing of proximal tooth surfaces: three-year clinical and radiographic follow-up. Caries Res 2008;42: 196.

5 Bonner BC, Clarkson JE, Dobbyn L, Khanna S: Slow-release fluoride devices for the control of dental decay. Cochrane Database Syst Rev 2006;18: CD005101.
6 Pessan JP, Al-Ibrahim NS, Buzalaf MA, Toumba KJ: Slow-release fluoride devices. J Appl Oral Sci 2008; 16:238–246.
7 Reynolds EC: Calcium phosphate-based remineralisation systems: scientific evidence? Aust Dent J 2008;53:268–273.
8 Papas A, Russell D, Singh M, Stack K, Kent R, Triol C, Winston A: Double blind clinical trial of remineralising dentifrice in the prevention of caries in radiation therapy patients. Gerodontology 1999;16: 2–10.
9 Papas A, Russell D, Singh M, Kent R, Triol C, Winston A: Caries clinical trial of a remineralising toothpaste in radiation patients. Gerodontolgy 2008;25:76–88.
10 Morgan MV, Adams GG, Bailey DL, Tsao CE, Fischman SL, Reynolds EC: The anticariogenic effect of sugar-free gum containing CPP-ACP nanocomplexes on approximal caries determined using digital bitewing radiographs. Caries Res 2008;42: 171–184.
11 Azarpazhooh A, Limeback H: Clinical efficacy of casein derivatives: a systematic review of the literature. J Am Dent Assoc 2008;139:915–924.
12 Azarpazhooh A, Limeback H: The application of ozone in dentistry: a systematic review of literature. J Dent 2008;36:104–116.
13 Brazelli M, McKenzie L, Fielding S, Fraser C, Clarkson J, Kilonzo M, Waugh N: Systematic review of the effectiveness and cost-effectiveness of Healozone for the treatment of occlusal pit/fissure caries and root caries. Health Technol Assess 2006;10:iii–iv, ix–80.
14 Goldin BR, Gorbach SL: Clinical indications for probiotics: an overview. Clin Infect Dis 2008;46 (suppl 2):S96–S100.
15 Garcia-Godoy F, Hicks MJ: Maintaining the integrity of the enamel surface: the role of the biofilm, saliva and preventive agents in enamel demineralisation and remineralisation. J Am Dent Assoc 2008; 139(suppl):25S–34S.
16 Twetman S, Steckson-Blicks C: Probiotics and oral health in children. Int J Paediatr Dent 2008;18:3–10.
17 Meurman JH, Stamatova I: Probiotics: contributions to oral health. Oral Dis 2007;13:443–451.
18 Hsu DJ, Darling CL, Lachica MM, Fried D: Nondestructive assessment of the inhibition of enamel demineralisation by CO_2 laser treatment using polarisation sensitive optical coherence tomography. J Biomed Opt 2008;13:054027.
19 Vlacic J, Meyers IA, Kim J, Walsh LJ: Laser-activated fluoride treatment of enamel against an artificial caries challenge: comparison of five wavelengths. Aust Dent J 2007;52:101–105.
20 Walsh LJ: The current status of laser applications in dentistry. Aust Dent J 2003;48:146–155.
21 Innes NP, Stirrups DR, Evans DJ, Hall N, Leggate M: A novel technique using preformed metal crowns for managing carious primary molars in general practice: a retrospective analysis. Br Dent J 2006; 200:451–454.
22 Innes NP, Evans DJ, Stirrups DR: The Hall technique: a randomised controlled clinical trial of a novel method of managing carious primary molars in general dental practice: acceptability of the technique and outcomes at 23 months. BMC Oral Health 2007;20:18.
23 The Japanese Ministry of Health and Labor: Report of National Survey of Oral Health in 2005. Tokyo, Association of Oral Health, 2007.
24 Pitts N: 'ICDAS': an international system for caries detection and assessment being developed to facilitate caries epidemiology, research and appropriate clinical management. Community Dent Health 2004;21:193–198.
25 Ismail AI, Sohn W, Tellez M, et al: Risk indicators for dental caries using the International Caries Detection and Assessment System. Community Dent Oral Epidemiol 2008;36:55–68.

C. Longbottom
Dental Health Services and Research Unit, University of Dundee
Mackenzie Building, Kirsty Semple Way
Dundee DD2 4BF (UK)
Tel. +44 1382 420064, Fax +44 1382 420051, E-Mail c.longbottom@cpse.dundee.ac.uk

Traditional Operative Treatment Options

D.N.J. Ricketts[a] · N.B. Pitts[b]

[a]Dundee Dental Hospital and School and [b]Dental Health Services and Research Unit, University of Dundee, Dundee, UK

Abstract

Operative intervention should be avoided, whenever possible, by adopting a preventive approach. Timely management of early caries can lead to arrest and possibly remineralization of the lesion rendering operative intervention unnecessary. The dentist must judge when the tooth tissue has become sufficiently demineralized to allow bacterial ingress leading to irreversible changes in the tissue. Once a decision has been made to restore a tooth, the clinician must decide, from a series of traditional *operative treatment options*, what materials should be used in the restoration and what preparation will achieve good retention and best preservation of tooth structure. With the development of new adhesive materials and a more conservative approach, a new era of minimally invasive dentistry has dawned. Improvements in the properties of composite materials have made them the choice for coronal aesthetic restorations: for posterior restorations involving load-bearing occlusal surfaces, amalgam is still the most commonly used material in UK dental practice; glass ionomer materials also have a place in minimally invasive dentistry – patterns of use differing in different counties. The numbers of studies investigating minimal caries removal are relatively limited; there are still scope and need for research in this field.

Copyright © 2009 S. Karger AG, Basel

When to Treat Operatively

A dentist's aim would be to avoid operative intervention wherever possible and to manage those patients at risk of developing caries, or those with early lesions, from a preventive point of view. However, if this preventive approach fails and the lesion progresses, a decision has to be made, somewhere along the continuum of the natural history of the disease process, to intervene operatively. Whilst this is a decision made by dentists on a daily basis, there is little substantiated evidence to say precisely when this decision should be taken. The problem being that, when this decision has been made, the patient will irreversibly enter the restorative cycle [1].

The first clinically visible sign of dental caries is a white-spot lesion. This develops as a result of biofilm formation on the surface of the tooth. The cariogenic organisms within this biofilm can ferment carbohydrates within the oral cavity, producing acids which diffuse into the tooth tissue resulting in demineralization. Management of caries at this stage simply involves regular disruption of the biofilm, preferably in the presence of fluoride. Such management can lead to arrest and possibly remineralization of the lesion, and operative intervention at this stage is completely contraindicated. Whilst some researchers have detected bacteria within early non-cavitated enamel lesions [2], they are in insufficient numbers to sustain lesion progression alone.

Some may use the enamel dentine junction as an operative threshold; however, the majority of these lesions will be non-cavitated on both the occlusal [3] and approximal surfaces [4, 5], the lesion still being driven by the bacterial biofilm on the surface of the tooth. So at what stage does the tooth tissue become so demineralized as to allow bacterial ingress to such a degree that the lesion becomes irreversible by plaque removal from the tooth surface alone?

As regards the occlusal surface, two clinical studies using microbiology to validate clinical and radiographic detection of caries have shown that it is only when the lesions are extensive enough to become radiographically visible that significant bacterial infection of the dentine occurs [3, 6]. Shallow occlusal dentine lesions are rarely seen on a bitewing radiograph, and it is only when a lesion extends into the middle third of dentine or deeper is it reliably detected [7]. Using a meticulous visual examination and classification system similar to the International Caries Detection and Assessment System (ICDAS) II, only dentine lesions scored as codes 3 or higher in the ICDAS II were significantly infected [6]. Interestingly, in approximately 40% of those scored as ICDAS II codes 3 and 4, no bacteria were cultured from the carious dentine, and it was only those that were radiographically visible that were infected. In a similar microbiological study on approximal lesions, it was shown that whilst non-cavitated dentine lesions were infected, they were significantly less infected than cavitated lesions. In the same study, it was shown that an approximal lesion was more likely to be cavitated if the radiolucency was deeper than 0.5 mm into dentine [8]. The majority of lesions radiographically just into dentine are non-cavitated [4].

Where Does This Evidence Fit with Previous Cavity or Lesion Classification Systems?

Towards the end of the 19th century, G.V. Black devised a classification system for recording cavity type based upon his detailed observations of carious lesions and cavity preparations (table 1). Perhaps surprisingly, this system is still used today by many teaching institutes around the world. It is based on which tooth surfaces the cavity involves; however, it does not take into consideration or detail the characteristics of the lesion that results in the cavity, such as the extent or severity of the lesion, and it does not inform the dentist as to 'when to restore'. It can also lead to what in modern times is considered to be overcutting of sound tooth tissue.

Table 1. Black's cavity classification

Black's cavity classification	Surfaces involved	Mount and Hume site code	Mount and Hume definition
Class I	Cavity involving the pits and fissures on the occlusal surface of posterior teeth	Site 1	Pits, fissures and enamel defects on occlusal surfaces of posterior teeth or other smooth surfaces (this site code would also include lesions in buccal pits and fissures)
Class II	Occluso-approximal cavity in posterior teeth	Site 2	Approximal enamel in relation to areas in contact with adjacent teeth
Class III	Approximal cavity in anterior teeth		
Class IV	Approximal cavity in anterior teeth also involving the incisal edge		
Class V	Buccal or lingual cervical cavity	Site 3	The cervical third of the crown or, following gingival recession, the exposed root

More recently, Mount et al. [9] have devised a new classification system to address these issues. The system is based on two parameters, namely the site of the lesion and the size of the lesion. The site parameter is a simplified version of Black's cavity classification (table 1). The size parameter is closely linked with the extent of the lesion, the treatment needs and the resultant cavity size when operative intervention is required (table 2). The ICDAS II classification [10] can be applied to individual tooth surfaces and fits well with the Mount and Hume site code. ICDAS II codes complement the Mount and Hume system by characterizing lesions in a way which is linked to histological depth. Further research in relation to ICDAS II on caries activity [see the chapter by Ekstrand et al., this vol., pp. 63–90] and the input of detection devices [see the chapters by Neuhaus et al., this vol., pp. 42–51 and 52–62] will build on the existing evidence and lead to a stronger evidence base for deciding upon the most appropriate operative treatment option at the right time. A recent and well-received proposal from the ICDAS Committee to the American Dental Association (fig. 1),

Table 2. Initial reconciliation of Mount-Hume and ICDAS classifications (for occlusal lesions)

Mount and Hume classification			ICDAS II
Size code	Size code definition	Size code proposed treatment	Corresponding codes
Size 0	The earliest lesion that can be identified as the initial stages of demineralization	Needs to be recorded but will be treated by eliminating the cause and should therefore not require further treatment	All codes 1 and 2 first visible change and distinct visible change
Size 1	Minimal surface cavitation with involvement of dentine just beyond treatment by remineralization alone	Some form of restoration is required to restore the smooth surface and prevent further plaque accumulation	Code 3 microcavitation on the occlusal surface if not radiographically visible suggested treatment: fissure seal
Size 2	Moderate involvement of dentine. Following cavity preparation remaining enamel is sound, well supported by dentine and not likely to fail under normal occlusal load	Conventional restoration remaining tooth sufficiently strong to support restoration	Code 4 undermining shadow on the occlusal surface if not radiographically visible suggested treatment: fissure seal
Size 3	The lesion is enlarged beyond moderate remaining tooth structure weakened to the extent that cusps or incisal ledges are …likely to fail if left exposed to occlusal load	The cavity needs to be further enlarged so that the restoration can be designed to provide support to the remaining tooth structure	Codes 5 and 6 extensive cavities exposing dentine

who have been consulting on a new caries classification, links the ICDAS detection codes grouped in pairs into 3 'stages' of caries to a simple Mount-Hume-like format which is colour coded. This system has the advantage of maintaining the ICDAS-defined link between the histological extent of the caries within the tooth.

Cavity Design

Once a decision has been made to restore a tooth, this does not render the patient disease free, and continued prevention is required to reduce the risk of developing

Sites of caries (1–4)	Stages of caries (0–3)			
	0 **No disease** ICDAS definition 0	1 **Initial** lesion ICDAS definitions 1 + 2	2 **Moderate** lesion ICDAS definitions 3 + 4	3 **Extensive** lesion ICDAS definition 5 + 6
1 Pit and fissure surfaces	1.0	1.1	1.2	1.3
2 Approximal surfaces	2.0	2.1	2.2	2.3
3 Cervical + smooth surfaces	3.0	3.1	3.2	3.3
4 Root surfaces	4.0	4.1	4.2	4.3

Fig. 1. Simplified format of a caries classification system for general practice and IT base level system suggested by the ICDAS Committee (following an American Dental Association workshop in 2008).

further primary caries or caries adjacent to the restoration. The initial stage of cavity preparation involves gaining access to the caries. For coronal caries, this usually involves removal of overlying enamel or restoration to gain access to the carious dentine. On the occlusal surface and free smooth surfaces buccally and lingually, this is straightforward; however, gaining access to approximal caries on posterior teeth can be from the buccal, lingual, fossa region (tunnel preparation) or through the marginal ridge. Where little gingival recession has taken place, the latter approach remains the most common. Once carious tissue has then been removed, the operator has to make a number of decisions and modify the cavity accordingly. The main decisions are what material is going to be used and what further tooth preparation is required to achieve retention (if necessary) and protect the remaining tooth structure.

Part of Black's work involved the observation of the location of initial carious lesions and the natural progression of the lesion. As such he was able to 'map out quite exactly the extent and boundaries of both the susceptible and immune areas on the surfaces of teeth'. This gave him an evidence base at the time for 'adequate cavity preparation and accurate restoration of lost structure, based on clinical observations', which 'generally prevented further extension of these carious lesions in the teeth treated'. So Black's principle for 'extension for prevention' was born, extending the cavity margins into so-called immune areas. On the occlusal surface of posterior teeth, this meant drilling out susceptible fissures beyond the area where caries had been removed, leaving the entire cavity margin in the 'immune' areas of the cuspal inclines. For approximal caries, the proximal box was extended buccally and lingually into the cleansable embrasure space, and the occlusal key was again cut, not only for resistance and retention form, but also to finish the cavity margins in less caries-susceptible sites. Such cavity preparation led to angular, undercut cavities and involved the removal of a large amount of sound tooth tissue. Mechanically retentive cavities were required as the materials used at the time, such as gold and amalgam, did not bond to the tooth tissue.

Black's principles of cavity design remained unquestioned for many years; however, with the development of new adhesive dental materials and a more conservative biological approach to caries removal and cavity design, a new era of minimally invasive dentistry dawned and was led by R.J. Elderton. In the mid 1980s, Elderton [11] took a new look at tooth preparation and suggested that only caries required removal and that extension for prevention was unnecessary. For occluso-approximal amalgam restorations on posterior teeth, retention for the proximal box could be provided by cutting buccal, lingual and gingival grooves in dentine. Extension onto the occlusal surface was only required when occlusal caries was present. This allowed a much more conservative approach to cavity design with a modern emphasis on the preservation of tooth tissue.

Restorative Materials Used

The properties of composite resin materials and the improved adhesion to enamel and dentine over the last 2 decades have made this the material of choice for coronal aesthetic restorations for anterior teeth or teeth within the smile line. Historically, glass-ionomer-based restorations produced superior bond strengths to dentine compared to the early dentine bonding agents used with composite resin, and this material was commonly used especially for the restoration of cavities prepared as a result of root caries. The glass ionomer materials release and take up fluoride, and these properties are commonly cited as a beneficial effect, especially in relation to the inhibition of secondary caries. However, a systematic review of the literature by Randal and Wilson [12] found no evidence to support or refute this hypothesis. This together with the fact that these materials are acid soluble and are seen by some as unsuitable for use on occlusal surfaces due to poor wear characteristics restrict their use as a definitive restoration in the UK. There is a variation of clinical opinion in other countries, and these materials are widely used.

For a posterior restoration involving the load-bearing occlusal surface, amalgam is still the material most commonly used in dental practice in the UK [13]. Whilst it is possible to bond amalgam into cavities, this is not routinely done and principles of cavity preparation that provide retention are still necessary. Unfounded health concerns over the use of mercury-containing amalgam and patient demands for tooth-coloured restorative materials have seen an increased use of composite materials in posterior teeth. This together with environmental concerns over waste mercury have led some dental schools to discontinue the teaching of dental amalgams, and dental schools throughout the UK have seen a reduction in the number of amalgam restorations placed in favour of composite resin [14]. Countries such as Norway and Sweden have also discontinued the use of dental amalgam in dental practice. This trend is likely to continue as the survival of composite resin restorations, demonstrated by the annual failure rates, is now comparable to that of amalgam restorations [15].

Impact of Composite Resin Use on Cavity Design

The use of composite resin has meant that following caries removal further cavity preparation is not required to gain retention for the restorations as the material bonds to the tooth tissue. This property also affords a heavily broken-down tooth some form of cusp re-enforcement. For less extensive cavities on the approximal or occlusal surface, the remaining fissure system no longer needs 'running out' with a dental bur to prevent caries occurring; instead, the unrestored aspect of the fissure can be fissure sealed. On the occlusal surface it has been suggested that any suspicious fissure could be investigated with a very small bur; if extensive caries is found, a conventional restoration will be required; however, if only a small amount of caries is present, the cavity can be restored with composite and a fissure sealant can be run over this and throughout the remaining fissure system. Some authors have suggested the use of glass ionomer in such cavities followed by fissure sealant application; however, the retention rate of the fissure sealant is inferior with this material. This has sometimes been referred to as a 'biopsy' technique and the restoration a preventive resin restoration. Given the importance of the bitewing radiograph and the ICDAS II criteria in determining the likelihood of bacterial infection within the dentine, as detailed in the first section of this chapter, this biopsy approach is not now considered necessary. If the lesion is non-cavitated and not visible radiographically, the lesion can either be managed with improved oral hygiene and monitored or fissure sealed. Fears of inadvertently sealing in caries in a stained fissure may be allayed, and this issue is discussed in the subsequent chapter by Ricketts and Pitts [this vol., pp. 174–187].

Minimally Invasive Dentistry – Tunnel Preparations

The concept of minimally invasive dentistry is not new, Simonsen [16] used it in 1987 in relation to the preventive resin restoration. The concept is maximum preservation of sound tooth tissue; however, it is often misinterpreted as early intervention and 'microdentistry' which is synonymous with overtreatment. Some may argue that on the occlusal surface a preventive resin restoration is unnecessary as these lesions could have been treated preventively if they were not visible on a bitewing radiograph.

To meet the needs of minimally invasive dentistry, the tunnel preparation was first described in the mid to late 1980s. It is well recognized that the marginal ridge of a posterior tooth offers strength to a tooth, its removal for access to caries on the approximal surface significantly weakens it. The tunnel preparation aimed to preserve the marginal ridge by accessing caries from the fossa area, tunnelling beneath the marginal ridge. The technique is clinically demanding and suffered a number of drawbacks, namely: access to the carious lesion is limited and as such caries removal is difficult and often incomplete; dentine is usually completely removed from beneath the marginal ridge enamel and the marginal ridge can fracture away; it is difficult to pack a restorative material into such a cavity without incorporating voids and to prepare such cavities tooth tissue is removed which is closer to the pulp running the risk of pulp horn exposure in a young patient. As such the tunnel preparation is rarely carried out in contemporary practice.

How Much Caries Do We Need to Remove?

Black wrote that 'generally when the cavity has been cut to form, no carious dentine will remain'. This judgement was made on a visual tactile basis, with removal of all discoloured dentine until hard dentine (to a sharp probe) was reached [17]. It is now known that demineralization of the dentine precedes discolouration which in turn precedes bacterial invasion [18]. Conventional cavity preparation has therefore been to gain access to the carious dentine and render the periphery of the cavity at the enamel-dentine junction caries and stain free. Pulpally, caries should be excavated using a hand excavator until hard but stained dentine is reached. The reasoning behind this is provided by Fusayama and Terashima [18], who, with the aid of a basic fuchsin dye, described two layers of carious dentine. In the outer zone the dentine is demineralized, the collagen denatured and there is bacterial invasion, hence the frequently used term 'infected zone'. In the inner zone, the dentine is demineralized but the collagen remains intact and there is minimal bacterial invasion. This inner zone is often referred to as the caries-affected zone, it is often stained and does not need to be removed during cavity preparation as it is capable of remineralization, only the outer infected zone needs to be removed which is not capable of remineralization.

Fusayama and Terashima [18] advocated the use of the caries detector dye to differentiate between these two layers and aid caries removal as the dye was purported to stain only the outer infected layer. Whilst the basic fuchsin dye used by them is no longer used due to its potential carcinogenicity, acid red dye and numerous other protein dyes have been used as caries detector dyes and are still advocated by some [19].

In two studies which have been carried out in undergraduate dental schools, the acid red dye has been applied to cavities which have been deemed to be caries free and complete by the operating student and supervising member of staff [20, 21]. In both studies, nearly 60% of cavities showed dye staining at the enamel-dentine junction, indicating that carious dentine had inadvertently been left. In a separate similar clinical study of 201 cavities where caries removal was thought to be complete and then the caries detector dye was applied, dentine samples were taken from dye-stained and dye-stain-free areas of the enamel-dentine junction and sent for microbiological analysis [22]. Low numbers of bacteria were cultured from both dye-stained and stain-free sites and there was no statistically significant difference between the two.

What would be the fate of such cavities if they had been filled with amalgam? The answer may lie in a laboratory study where such teeth were restored with amalgam and thermocycled in tea and chlorhexidine [23]. In areas at the enamel-dentine junction the dentine had picked up stain, and histological examination revealed that this corresponded to the areas of demineralization or residual caries. Clinical studies would support the fact that hard and stained dentine can be left at the enamel-dentine junction, because these areas are minimally infected and this is now what is taught in a number of dental schools. Peripheral stain may however need to be removed under tooth-coloured restorations from an aesthetic point of view.

Strength of Evidence for Traditional Operative Management

Traditional operative intervention has changed very little since Black and is still managed as if the carious lesion was dental gangrene. The lesion is excised, albeit more conservatively, and a prosthetic restoration placed. The management is based on what the dental profession regards as best clinical practice and clinical experience. Restoration survival data allow the annual failure rate of restorations to be calculated; however, fewer amalgam restorations are now being placed, and dental material science and manufacturers introduce newer material at a rate that makes a sound evidence base difficult to obtain; by the time a carefully planned prospective randomised controlled trial of sufficient duration is executed and published, the material has often been superseded.

References

1. Elderton RJ: Clinical studies concerning re-restoration of teeth. Adv Dent Res 1990;4:4–9.
2. Parolo CC, Maltz M: Microbial contamination of noncavitated caries lesions: a scanning electron microscopic study. Caries Res 2006;40:536–541.
3. Ricketts DN, Kidd EA, Beighton D: Operative and microbiological validation of visual, radiographic and electronic diagnosis of occlusal caries in noncavitated teeth judged to be in need of operative care. Br Dent J 1995;179:214–220.
4. Hintze H, Wenzel A, Danielsen B: Behaviour of approximal carious lesions assessed by clinical examination after tooth separation and radiography: a 2.5-year longitudinal study in young adults. Caries Res 1999;33:415–422.
5. Lunder N, von der Fehr FR: Approximal cavitation related to bite-wing image and caries activity in adolescents. Caries Res 1996;30:143–147.
6. Ricketts DN, Ekstrand KR, Kidd EA, Larsen T: Relating visual and radiographic ranked scoring systems for occlusal caries detection to histological and microbiological evidence. Oper Dent 2002;27:231–237.

7 Ricketts DN, Kidd EA, Smith BG, Wilson RF: Clinical and radiographic diagnosis of occlusal caries: a study in vitro. J Oral Rehabil 1995;22:15–20.
8 Ratledge DK, Kidd EA, Beighton D: A clinical and microbiological study of approximal carious lesions. 1. The relationship between cavitation, radiographic lesion depth, the site-specific gingival index and the level of infection of the dentine. Caries Res 2001;35: 3–7.
9 Mount GJ, Tyas JM, Duke ES, Hume WR, Lasfargues JJ, Kaleka R: A proposal for a new classification of lesions of exposed tooth surfaces. Int Dent J 2006; 56:82–91.
10 ICDAS – International Caries Detection and Assessment System. www.icdas.org.
11 Elderton RJ: New approaches to cavity design with special reference to the class II lesion. Br Dent J 1984;157:421–427.
12 Randal RC, Wilson NH: Glass-ionomer restoratives: a systematic review of a secondary caries treatment effect. J Dent Res 1999;78:628–637.
13 Burke FJ, McHugh S, Hall AC, Randall RC, Widstrom E, Forss H: Amalgam and composite use in UK general dental practice in 2001. Br Dent J 2003;194:613–618.
14 Lynch CD, Shortall AC, Stewardson D, Tomson PL, Burke FJ: Teaching posterior composite resin restorations in the United Kingdom and Ireland: consensus views of teachers. Br Dent J 2007;203:183–187.
15 Hickel R, Manhart J: Longevity of restorations in posterior teeth and reasons for failure. J Adhes Dent 2001;3:45–64.
16 Simonsen RJ: The preventive resin restoration: a minimally invasive, non-metallic restoration. Compendium 1987;8:428–430.
17 Black GV: Operative Dentistry. II. Technical Procedures, ed 7. London, Kimpton, 1936, pp 140–141.
18 Fusayama T, Terashima S: Differentiation of two layers of carious dentin by staining. J Dent Res 1972; 51:866.
19 Goracci G, Ferrari M: Direct posterior restorations – techniques for effective placement; in Roulet J-F, Wilson NHF, Fuzzi M (eds): Advances in Operative Dentistry. London, Quintessence Publishing, 2001, vol 1: Contemporary clinical practice.
20 Kidd EA, Joyston-Bechal S, Smith MM, Allan R, Howe L, Smith SR: The use of a caries detector dye in cavity preparation. Br Dent J 1989;167:132–134.
21 Anderson MH, Charbeneau GT: A comparison of digital and optical criteria for detecting carious dentin. J Prosthet Dent 1985;53:643–646.
22 Kidd EA, Joyston-Bechal S, Beighton D: The use of a caries detector dye during cavity preparation: a microbiological assessment. Br Dent J 1993;175:312–313.
23 Kidd EA, Joyston-Bechal S, Smith MM: Staining of residual caries under freshly-packed amalgam restorations exposed to tea/chlorhexidine in vitro. Int Dent J 1990;40:219–224.

David Ricketts
Dundee Dental Hospital and School
Park Place
Dundee DD1 4HR (UK)
Tel./Fax +44 1382 635984, E-Mail d.n.j.ricketts@dundee.ac.uk

Novel Operative Treatment Options

D.N.J. Ricketts[a] · N.B. Pitts[b]

[a]Dundee Dental Hospital and School and [b]Dental Health Services and Research Unit, University of Dundee, Dundee, UK

Abstract

There are an increasing number of more novel options available for operative intervention. This chapter outlines a series of *operative treatment options* which are available to the modern clinician to select from once a decision has been made to treat a carious lesion operatively. A series of *novel methods of caries removal* have been described; including chemomechanical caries removal, air abrasion, sono-abrasion, polymer rotary burs and lasers. There are also *novel approaches to ensure complete caries removal* and *novel approaches for the management of deep caries*. A novel question increasingly asked by clinicians is: does all the caries need to be removed? Operative management options here include: therapeutic fissure sealants, ultraconservative caries removal, stepwise excavation and the Hall technique. In conclusion, there is now a growing wealth of evidence that questions the traditional methods of caries removal and restoring the tooth. In parallel, there is a growing movement exploring the merits of therapeutically sealing caries into the tooth. This philosophy is alien to many of today's dentists and, until further randomized controlled trials are carried out in primary care, prudent caution must be exercised with this promising approach. Research is required into techniques which will allow monitoring of sealed caries to detect any rare, but insidious, failures. These novel techniques are an alternative way of managing the later stages of the caries process from a sounder biological basis and have marked potential benefits to patients from treatment, pain and outcome perspectives.

Copyright © 2009 S. Karger AG, Basel

Once a decision has been made to treat a carious lesion operatively, traditional teaching of cavity preparation has been to gain access to the caries with a high-speed bur, then change to a slow handpiece with a round bur to remove peripheral caries and then to an excavator to cleave away pulpal dentine caries. In a vital tooth, the pulp and dentine are inextricably linked by virtue of the odontoblastic process, dentine is therefore a vital tissue, and to prepare a cavity by excising the caries usually requires a local anaesthetic. The heat generated by an inadequately cooled high-speed handpiece, the vibration from a slow handpiece and overjudicious caries removal can all irreversibly damage the dental pulp. Traditional teaching has been to selectively remove only the outer, infected layer of carious dentine [see the chapter by Ricketts and Pitts, this vol., pp. 164–173], leaving the inner caries-affected zone. However, use of dental burs has been shown to be the least selective method to differentiate between the two layers and can lead to overpreparation of the cavity; only an excavator should be used pulpally to remove caries [1]. A series of alternative methods of caries removal which might resolve some of these issues have been described.

Novel Methods of Caries Removal

Chemomechanical Caries Removal – Carisolv

The idea for the use of chemicals to assist in the mechanical removal of dental caries was first suggested in the middle of the 1970s and led to production of the Caridex system in the 1980s. The system required the use of a reservoir for the chemicals to be used, a heater and a pump, which pumped the solution to a handpiece applicator via a tube. The solution assisted in the loosening of carious dentine by chlorinating the collagen, facilitating its removal with specially designed applicators which were used with a scraping action. A series of factors, including the complex equipment required, the large volumes of liquid used per cavity preparation (100–500 ml) and the increased time the technique required as compared to conventional cavity preparation led to its demise as a routine tool for clinical practice.

A number of the problems associated with the Caridex system have been overcome with the more recently introduced Carisolv system. The delivery of Carisolv has been simplified to the contents of 2 syringes which are mixed when required. The first syringe contains sodium hypochlorite (0.5%) and the second a combination of glutamic acid, lysine, leucine, carboxymethylcellulose, sodium chloride, sodium hydroxide and a red dye. The isotonic gel produced is applied to the cavity and causes proteolytic degradation of the already partially broken-down collagen in the outer zone of carious dentine. Specially designed hand instruments are again used to abrade the altered dentine. Intermittent rinsing using the 3-in-1 syringe and reapplication of the gel are required to remove the dentine particles from the cavity. Once mixed, the Carisolv gel remains active for up to 20 min and, because it is alkaline, it does not cause demineralization of sound dentine. As a result, overpreparation of the cavity is prevented and the use of local anaesthetic can often be avoided. Due to the way in which the carious dentine is removed, the cavity is left smear layer free, providing an optimum surface for the modern generation of dentine bonding agents used with composite resin restorative materials.

Air Abrasion

Air abrasion has been described as a pseudomechanical method of cutting tooth tissue using fine alumina particles, 27.5 µm in diameter, which are ejected out of a nozzle tip under air pressure. The hardness and kinetic energy of the particles effectively abrade the carious tooth tissue away. Some of the variables that influence the cutting ability of the air abrasion stream are the air pressure at the nozzle tip, the diameter of the nozzle tip and the distance the nozzle tip is from the tooth tissue being cut. Unlike a dental bur which is end and side cutting, air abrasion is end cutting only, and, unlike a dental bur in a handpiece, there is no sensory feedback as to the hardness of the tissues being cut. As a result, there is no discrimination between carious and sound tooth tissue and there is a significant risk of overpreparing the cavity; in fact, air abrasion with alumina cuts harder sound tissue more efficiently than softer carious tissue [2]. This, together with the fact that the technique creates a cloud of dust, with possible problems associated with inhalation and cross-infection control, has made it a technique for cavity preparation with limited popularity. Its use for 'examining' stained fissures should be treated cautiously as overcutting of sound fissures or arrested initial lesions may result.

Sono-Abrasion

This technique consists of specially designed diamond-coated tips used in air-scaler handpieces, the high-frequency sonic oscillations allowing dental hard tissue removal. Little research has been published on this technique for caries removal and cavity preparation. However, that which has been published has suggested that its use could lead to inadequate caries removal when compared to the natural autofluorescent signal from carious dentine [1].

Polymer Rotary Burs – Smartprep, SS White

Smartprep polymer burs are a relatively recent and novel introduction for selective dentine caries removal. These polymer burs are designed to only remove the softened outer zone of carious dentine; as sound harder dentine is approached, the flutes or paddles on the bur become blunt and unable to remove further tooth tissue. Published data on the use of these burs is very limited; 3 in vitro studies were found in a Pubmed literature search in December 2008. One study showed that significantly less sound dentine is removed with the Smartprep burs compared to a stainless-steel round bur [3]. Based on time for caries removal, no difference was found between Smartprep burs and conventional tungsten carbide burs [4, 5]. However, based upon residual caries left following cavity preparation, one study found no difference between the two bur types [4], and another found that the Smartprep burs left significantly more caries than the carbide bur [5]; whether this would be clinically significant is a more important question to ask, and more information is needed.

Lasers

Lasers are named after and are characteristic of the element from which they are derived following stimulated quantum transitions within the orbiting electron shells. The light produced from each element is essentially of the same wavelength (monochromatic), and its properties will to a large degree be dependent on its wavelength, duration of exposure and the properties of the tissues on which it is used. Laser light is transmitted into the target tissues and its penetration will depend on the laser's wavelength. The light energy absorbed by the tissues is then transferred into heat which could be a major disadvantage when caries removal and maintenance of a healthy pulp are concerned.

The lasers which have been mainly used in caries removal and cavity preparation are based on erbium, namely Er:YAG (erbium:yttrium-aluminium-garnet) and Er,Cr:YSGG (eribium-chromium:yttrium-selenium-gallium-garnet) lasers. These lasers have a wavelength of 2.94 and 2.78 μm, respectively, and are conveyed in a pulsed waveform which delivers high-intensity energy in small interrupted bursts. The main advantages cited for the erbium lasers are that they have a shallow depth of penetration into the tooth tissue and are therefore unlikely to cause pulpal damage, the local heat generated causes little localized cracking and a cavity following laser ablation is left without a smear layer which again is optimal for dentine bonding [6].

One major drawback of laser cavity reparation, as with air abrasion, is that there is no sensory feedback to the clinician to know when caries has been completely removed. However, recent research would suggest that this can be overcome by using laser ablation of tooth tissue in conjunction with a laser fluorescence feedback system of an excitation wavelength of 655 nm to control the laser cutting [7, 8]. When a threshold of 7 was used by these authors to cease caries removal, complete removal of all infected carious dentine was found.

A review of the literature on lasers has shown that the public's expectation of their dentists' use of lasers in dental practice is high; however, there are few benefits to be gained in caries removal and cavity preparation over and above that of conventional techniques currently accepted [6]. Whilst patients might prefer the possibilities that the use of lasers may afford, namely the use of no local anaesthetic and the lack of the vibration and sound of a dental drill, the added cost and bulk of the equipment needed may very well offset this demand.

Novel Approaches Used to Ensure Complete Caries Removal

The novel caries removal techniques described in this chapter and the traditional operative intervention in the preceding chapter have all aimed at either complete caries removal or removal of the outer infected zone of carious dentine, leaving the inner caries-affected zone pulpally. To ensure that this goal is met, some clinicians still use caries detector dyes; however, it is clear from the preceding chapter that such dyes not only stain the outer infected zone of caries, but also the demineralized inner zone of caries or less mineralized dentine pulpally and at the enamel-dentine junction [9]. Dye staining is therefore not a good indicator of bacterial invasion of the dentine, and its use can lead to overpreparation of a cavity and it should therefore be avoided.

To ensure that all infected carious dentine is removed (if this is required), the use of laser detection devices has been suggested [10, 11]. One such device, the DIAGNOdent, operates at an excitation wavelength of 655 nm, which leads to increased fluorescence from bacterial by-products, namely porphyrins or chromophores [12, 13]; the presence of bacteria alone has been shown not to lead to such a fluorescence [13]. The principle is therefore based upon the fact that the bacterial porphyrins will lie adjacent to the bacteria and not diffuse into deeper tissues unlike the bacterially produced acid. If the latter were the case or if the dentine were darkly stained, higher laser fluorescence readings could lead to overpreparation of the cavity. In addition, it has been suggested that readings are unreliable in deeper cavities closer to the pulp [14]. The use of such devices in cavity preparation is therefore questionable, especially in light of the subsequent arguments to be presented below.

Management of Deep Caries

Traditional operative management of caries as described previously poses a major threat to the pulp in deeper cavities where complete caries removal leads to a thinner remaining dentine thickness (RDT). It is clear that when the RDT is reduced, the risk of pulp pathology and loss of vitality is higher [15]. The RDT has been shown in a recent ex vivo model to be the most important operative variable which can lead to pulpal injury when compared to the absence of water coolant during cavity preparation, the speed of the bur and hence the heat generated, potential harmful effects from cavity conditioners and the filling material used to restore the cavity [16]. It has also been shown that in symptomless teeth with deep lesions the risk of exposing the pulp is relatively high: 40% risk in permanent teeth [17] and 53% in primary teeth [18].

Pulpal exposure in teeth with no clinical symptoms, no radiographic evidence of pathology and an exposure which is in relation to a vital pulp which stops bleeding readily has traditionally been managed with a direct pulp cap using calcium hydroxide. Assessment of the success rate of this technique is difficult due to a lack of standardization of technique and the fact that most studies have been carried out on traumatic exposures of previously healthy teeth. In a study of 123 teeth that had received direct pulp caps following a carious exposure, the success rate at 5 years was 37% and at 10 years only 13% [19]. The predictability of this technique with traditional materials has therefore been questioned; however, more recent data on the use of mineral trioxide aggregate have suggested a more reliable outcome [20].

Measurement of Remaining Dentine Thickness

In view of the injury to the pulp and the fact that its long-term health is severely compromised when the RDT is reduced and when the pulp is exposed, researchers have investigated methods of measuring the RDT to ensure that it is not compromised during cavity preparation. In 1994 an ultrasonic micrometer was investigated in vitro on dentine discs, extracted human teeth and in vivo on dog teeth. In both settings, strong relationships were found between ultrasonically measured RDT and the actual RDT [21]. Despite this early promise, little further work has been carried out.

Electrical resistance measurements have also been used to indicate the RDT. This was initially suggested by Yoshida et al. [22] in 1989, but it was concluded that measurement errors would make it difficult to estimate the RDT. In 2007 this method was re-evaluated with a device called the Prepometer (Hager & Werken, Duisburg, Germany) [23]. In this study measurements were made in cavities which were cut in teeth due for extraction, allowing actual RDT to be measured. Whilst the reproducibility of the device was found to be good, the relationship between the resistance measurements and actual RDT was poor. This is understandable, as it is not only the RDT that will dictate the electrical resistance, but also the level of dentine mineralization and tubular sclerosis that might have taken place.

Methods of measuring RDT have, to date, not been successful, and if the subsequent view on conservative cavity preparation and caries removal is adopted, further research in this area may be superfluous.

Does Caries Need to Be Removed?

The traditional and novel management of caries described so far in this and the preceding chapter has been based on what has been regarded previously as best clinical practice, but despite our understanding of the carious process, its aetiology and histopathology, it is still managed like a gangrenous limb: complete excision and replacement with a prosthesis. Despite a completely different aetiology to gangrene, the operative management of dental caries in clinical practice has remained essentially unchanged and unquestioned over the last 2 centuries. However, in 1993 Hume [24] questioned the need for a change in caries management based 'on the structure and behaviour of the caries lesion'.

Once a carious lesion has cavitated and/or extended into the dentine to such a degree that the dentine has become heavily infected, the bacteria within the lesion still obtain most of their substrate from dietary sugars within the oral cavity, although it is possible for a smaller amount of substrate to be obtained from tissue fluids which permeate outwards from the pulp. Preventing the bacteria within the lesion from obtaining this substrate has been shown to have a profound effect in 4 types of studies. These are fissure sealant studies, ultraconservative caries removal studies, stepwise excavation studies and studies on the Hall technique, where the common principle is to seal the carious lesion into the tooth and isolate it from the oral cavity and dietary sugars.

Fissure Sealant Studies

The possibility of using fissure sealants over carious fissures as a therapeutic intervention was suggested in the mid to late 1970s by two groups of workers led by Handelman and Mertz-Fairhurst [25–27]. In these studies both groups showed that by sealing dentine caries into the tooth, the number of viable organisms within decreased significantly. This was found to be most profound in the first 2 weeks after sealing with a continued gradual reduction in organisms thereafter [25]. Acid etching alone, in preparation for the fissure sealant, was found to reduce the number of organisms by up to 75%, and after 12 months of being fissure sealed the number of viable organisms within the carious dentine was found to have fallen by 99.9% [28]. Clinical and radiographic observations of sealed lesions after 1 year [27] and 2 years [29] have shown that there is no evidence of caries progression and in the latter study there is even a suggestion of lesion regression. During the study periods, none of the cited studies report any signs or symptoms of pulp pathology, and in those teeth where the fissure sealant was lost, little effect on the radiographic severity scoring was found [28]. This may have been due to too short a duration following sealant loss and reassessment for lesion progression to occur, or it may be due to the fact that whilst the bulk of the sealant was lost, tags of sealant may remain in the base of the fissure ensuring a continued seal.

It is known that the retention rates of resin-based fissure sealants are superior to other dental materials, and retention rates of fissure sealants placed in carious fissures have been reported to be comparable to those placed in sound fissures over a 2-year period [30]. A recent Cochrane systematic review has shown that the complete retention rate of resin fissure sealants after 1 year is 79–92%, after 2 years 61–85%, after 4 years 52% and after 9 years 39% [31]. In addition to complete loss of fissure sealant, sealants undergo partial loss, partial debonding and wear. If caries is fissure sealed into a tooth, regular recall is therefore required to monitor the integrity of the fissure sealant and, where necessary, replace or repair. Failure to do so could lead to progression of the lesion.

Ultraconservative Caries Removal

Whilst sealing caries into the tooth has been shown to have the potential to arrest the carious process, fissure sealant durability is a possible problem. Ultraconservative caries removal and restoration with a more durable composite restoration addresses this problem. Ultraconservative caries removal was described by Mertz-Fairhurst et al. [32] and involves cutting a 45- to 60-degree bevel in the fissure enamel to achieve at least a 1-mm-wide rim of sound enamel around the entire periphery of the small cavity removing any crumbly opaque carious enamel; no attempt was made to remove any dentine caries. The cavity was then etched, rinsed and dried and a good etch pattern confirmed before restoring with a composite resin. Following this, any unfilled fissure was fissure sealed following a further etch, rinse and drying procedure.

In the split-mouth randomized controlled trial by Mertz-Fairhurst et al., patients were screened for paired posterior teeth with obvious cavitated occlusal lesions which had a radiolucency visible on bitewing radiographs but no deeper than half the way through the dentine. In total, 123 patients with 156 pairs of study teeth were recruited into the study. One of each pair was randomly allocated to the test, ultraconservative caries removal group, the other control tooth was then further randomly allocated to either (a) a complete caries removal group where the cavity was filled with amalgam and the remaining fissure system was sealed or to (b) a complete caries removal group where the cavity was extended into the remaining sound fissure (extension for prevention) and then restored with amalgam. Outcomes for this study have been published for time points from 6 months to 2, 3, 4, 5, 6, 9 and 10 years [32–38].

Compared to the numbers recruited, the proportion of teeth in each group available for analysis at each time interval is given in figure 1. The general drop at 6 years or more is likely to be due to patients lost to recall (no reason given) and the small differences between the test and two control groups at each recall interval is due to teeth being lost to the study because of failure. Figure 2 gives the proportion of teeth lost to failure (related to the restoration) after each time interval compared to baseline; this therefore represents cumulative failure. No statistically significant difference was found at 10 years between the survival of the ultraconservative restoration and the amalgam restoration which was extended for prevention; however, a difference was detected between the ultraconservative restoration and the sealed amalgam, with the amalgam outperforming the composite restoration. Failures were due to loss of marginal integrity to restorations, loss of sealant, loss of restoration and wear; no failures were reported due to signs or symptoms of pulp pathology, and all restoration failures were therefore retrievable.

Stepwise Excavation

Stepwise excavation is a technique which has been described with the main aim to reduce the risk of pulpal exposure during caries removal in teeth with deep carious lesions. In this technique caries is progressively removed in two separate procedures 4–12 months apart. In the first procedure, access to the dentine caries is gained and peripheral caries is completely removed at the enamel-dentine junction or cervical floor of a proximal lesion. On the pulpal floor of the cavity, no attempt is made to remove soft carious dentine, provided that there is sufficient space to place an adequate calcium hydroxide lining and restoration. It is important that the peripheral

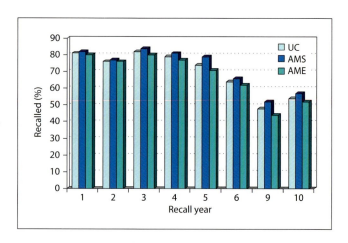

Fig. 1. Compared to the numbers recruited originally, the proportion of teeth in each group available for analysis at each time interval in the split-mouth randomized controlled trial of Mertz-Fairhurst et al.'s [32–38]. UC = Ultraconservative composite; AMS = amalgam sealed; AME = amalgam extended.

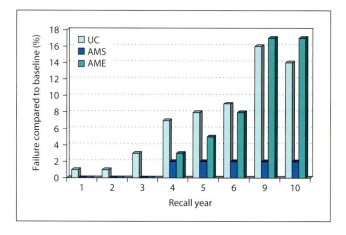

Fig. 2. Proportion of teeth lost due to failure (related to the restoration) after each time interval compared to baseline (cumulative failure) in the split-mouth randomized controlled trial of Mertz-Fairhurst et al. [32–38]. UC = Ultraconservative composite; AMS = amalgam sealed; AME = amalgam extended.

caries removal and restoration placed achieve a hermetic seal to the carious dentine left behind. Four to 12 months later, the restoration is removed and the residual pulpal caries is then carefully excavated.

A stepwise excavation study on sealed caries has shown that when the cavity is re-entered the residual caries becomes harder and drier in consistency and darker in colour, features which are consistent with lesion arrest [39, 40]. In a separate study, where subtraction radiography was used to monitor changes in the depth of the radiolucency beneath restorations where incomplete caries removal had taken place, there was no evidence of lesion progression; to the contrary, there was reduction in radiolucency depth in 38% of sealed lesions consistent with remineralization [41]. In this study the lesions were monitored for 36–45 months, and where the radiolucency depth decreased, it did so in the first 6 months with little evidence thereafter.

Microbial analysis of the caries at the end of the first excavation and at the start of the second has shown that there is a decrease in the number of viable organisms present [39], a result consistent with those of Paddick et al. [42], who have also shown that there is a reduction in the microbial diversity. In this stepwise excavation study, lactobacillus counts were reduced to zero after sealing in the dentine caries, and whilst the proportional contribution of streptococcus species increased, there was a reduction in the range of species from 8 to 3, with only *Streptococcus oralis, intermedius* and *mitis* being cultured at the second excavation. Of the Gram-positive pleomorphic rods whose proportional contribution fell, only *Actinomyces naeslundii* survived. Those organisms that survive are those capable of breaking down pulpal glycoproteins into sugars for metabolism, and these organisms are not particularly associated with active carious lesions. In response to the carious process the pulp-dentine complex lays down reactionary dentine and peritubular dentine, the latter leading to tubular sclerosis. These processes further reduce the nutrient supply to the organisms that do survive such a stressed environment, and eventually these too are likely to die [25].

Systematic Review: Complete versus Ultraconservative Removal of Decayed Tissue

Whilst the clinical studies cited support the fact that caries removal is not necessary when a restoration or fissure sealant can be placed which provides and maintains a seal between the residual caries and the oral cavity, the strongest level of evidence is provided by prospective randomized controlled trials. A Cochrane systematic review of the literature was therefore carried out to search for such trials comparing ultraconservative caries removal with complete caries removal [43]. The Cochrane Oral Health Group Trials Register, Cochrane Central Register of Controlled Trials, Medline, Pubmed and Embase databases were all searched, and initially 529 titles and abstracts were read, with 49 articles potentially meeting the inclusion criteria. These full papers were all read and finally only 4 publications could be included. The included papers were 2 stepwise excavation studies, 1 on permanent teeth [17] and 1 on primary teeth [18], and 2 studies where caries was sealed permanently into the teeth [33, 44].

The Cochrane review enabled data to be collected from 339 patients and 604 teeth (538 available for analysis). Data were obtained from 3 studies at 1 year for comparison, and at this time period, no problems were reported in relation to signs and symptoms of pulp pathology or retention rates of the restorations. The most striking result was in relation to pulpal exposure during caries removal in the stepwise excavation studies. Complete caries removal in permanent teeth with deep lesions resulted in exposure of the pulp in 40% of cases compared to 0% after the first stage of stepwise excavation and 17.5% when the teeth were re-entered [17]. Similarly in primary teeth, complete caries removal resulted in exposure of the pulp in 53% of cases compared to 0% after the first stage of stepwise excavation and 15% when the teeth were re-entered [18].

It is clear that sealing caries into the teeth allowed for pulp-dentine complex reactions to take place, significantly reducing the risk of pulpal exposure. In the study by Leksell et al. [17], the lesions were re-entered after 8–24 weeks, a shorter period compared to that recommended by Bjørndal et al. [39]. In a separate practice-based study, when lesions were re-entered after 2–19 months (median 6 months), fewer exposures (5%, 6 out of 94 teeth) were experienced on re-entering [40], and in a similar study by Maltz et al. [45], when lesions were re-entered after 6–7 months, only 6% led to exposure or pulp pathology (2 out of 32). Sealing for a longer period still may allow further remineralization of the dentine caries and pulp-dentine complex reactions to take place and reduce the risk of pulpal exposure on re-entering even further. Some researchers have also questioned whether re-entry is required [43, 46]. In a study where 32 teeth which had undergone the first stage of stepwise excavation and were re-entered simply to take a dentine sample for microbial analysis and then immediately resealed without further caries removal and followed for 36–45 months, cumulative failures amounted to 16%: 1 (3%) developed pulp necrosis, 1 (3%) pulp was exposed on re-entry, 2 restorations fractured and 1 restoration was replaced at a different clinic [41]. This study would give support to the argument that re-entry is not required as failures were few, one of which resulted from the fact that the cavity was re-entered.

Hall Technique

The final technique which questions the need for caries removal is the Hall technique used to manage carious primary teeth by Innes et al. [47]. In this technique, primary molar teeth with caries affecting 2 or more surfaces are restored with a preformed stainless-steel crown. However, unlike the traditionally taught technique, no caries removal takes place and no tooth preparation is carried out, the crown is simply filled with a glass ionomer cement and with either finger pressure or the child's occlusal force, the crown is cemented onto the tooth. In a retrospective analysis of 975 teeth with approximal caries into dentine in 259 children (mean age 5 years at placement) managed in such a way showed that the probability of the crown survival for 3 years was 73.4% and the likelihood of the tooth surviving for this period without being extracted was 86% [47]. This success rate compares favourably with conventional restorations where the 3-year success rate has been estimated to be 50–93% depending on the restorative material chosen [47].

Whilst this procedure was carried out in primary care by a general dental practitioner as part of routine management of child patients, no data are given on the longevity of that practitioner's conventional restorations; in addition, only one operator was involved, therefore questioning its extrapolation to other dentists and populations. To address this, Innes et al. [48] devised in a further study a prospective randomized controlled split-mouth trial to compare the Hall technique with conventional restorations that the participating dentists would normally place. In all, 17 general dental practitioners took part who recruited 132 children. In total, 128 Hall crowns and 128 conventional restorations were placed with 124 from each group available for analysis at 2 years. At placement the child, carer or parent and dentist were given questionnaires to assess any discomfort from and the acceptability of both procedures. The Hall technique was found to cause less discomfort at placement than the conventional restoration and was favoured by the majority of children, and their carer/parent and dentist.

Signs or symptoms of pulp pathology were regarded as major failures, and minor failures were loss of restoration or caries progression. At 2 years there were only 3 major failures in the Hall group (2%) and 19 in the control group (15%) [48]. Minor failures occurred in 6 of the Hall group (5%) and 57 of the control group (46%). The Hall technique was therefore found to be more acceptable to all involved than conventional dentistry and was accompanied by significantly fewer major and minor failures; importantly, there was also significantly less pain reported in the Hall group.

In conclusion, there is a growing wealth of evidence that questions the traditional methods of caries removal and restoring the tooth. In parallel, there is a growing movement exploring the merits of therapeutically sealing caries into the tooth. The stressed environment the bacteria are then subjected to leads to a slowing and arrest of the lesion activity in dentine. This philosophy is alien to today's dentists, and until further randomized controlled trails similar to those in the recent Cochrane review [43] are carried out in primary care, assessing the success and acceptability of the sealing techniques, little change will take place and prudent caution must be exercised with this promising approach. Dentists are concerned that if the seal in relation to these techniques breaks down, the lesion will progress rapidly. As with conventional restorations, review and assessment of the integrity of the sealed restorations will be of importance as will appropriate action taken when any failure occurs. The development of approximal sealants is a further innovation [49]. Research will also be required into techniques which will allow monitoring of sealed caries to detect any rare insidious failures; subtraction radiography is one possibility [50]. These novel techniques are an alternative way of managing the later stages of the caries process from a sounder biological basis and have marked potential benefits to patients from treatment, pain and outcome perspectives.

References

1 Banerjee A, Kidd EA, Watson TF: In vitro evaluation of five methods of carious dentine excavation. Caries Res 2000;34:144–150.
2 Paolinelis G, Watson TF, Banerjee A: Microhardness as a predictor of sound and carious dentine removal using alumina air abrasion. Caries Res 2006;40:292–295.
3 Hauman CH, Kuzmanovic DV: An evaluation of polymer rotary instruments' ability to remove healthy, non-carious dentine. Eur J Prosthodont Restor Dent 2007;15:77–80.
4 Meller C, Welk A, Zeligowski T, Splieth C: Comparison of dentin caries excavation with polymer and tungsten carbide burs. Quintessence Int 2007; 38:565–569.

5 Dammaschke T, Rodenberg TN, Schäfer, Ott KH: Efficiency of the polymer bur Smartprep compared with conventional tungsten carbide bud bur in dentin caries excavation. Oper Dent 2006;31:256–260.
6 Dederich DN, Bushick RD, ADA Council on Scientific Affairs and Division of Science: Lasers in dentistry: separating science from hype. J Am Dent Assoc 2004;135:204–212.
7 Eberhard J, Eisenbeiss AK, Braun A, Hedderich J, Jepsen S: An evaluation of selective caries removal by a fluorescence feedback-controlled Er:YAG laser in vitro. Caries Res 2005;39:496–504.
8 Jepsen S, Acil Y, Perschel T, Kargas K, Eberhard J: Biochemical and morphological analysis of dentin following selective caries removal with a fluorescence-controlled Er:YAG laser. Laser Surg Med 2008;40:350–357.
9 McComb D: Caries-detector dyes – how accurate and useful are they? J Can Dent Assoc 2000;66:195–198.
10 Lennon AM: Fluorescence-aided caries excavation (FACE) compared to conventional method. Oper Dent 2003;28:341–345.
11 Lennon AM, Buchalla W, Switsalski L, Stookey GK: Residual caries detection using visible fluorescence. Caries Res 2002;36:315–319.
12 König K, Flemming G, Hibst R: Laser-induced autofluorescence spectroscopy of dental caries. Cell Mol Biol (Noisy-le-Grand) 1998;44:1293–1300.
13 Banerjee A, Gilmour A, Kidd E, Watson T: Relationship between *Streptococcus mutans* and the autofluorescence of carious dentin. Am J Dent 2004; 17:233–236.
14 Krause F, Braun A, Eberhard J, Jepsen S: Laser fluorescence measurements compared to electrical resistance of residual dentine in excavated cavities in vivo. Caries Res 2007;41:135–140.
15 Wisithphrom K, Murray PE, About I, Windsor LJ: Interactions between cavity preparation and restoration events and their effects on pulp vitality. Int J Periodontics Restorative Dent 2006;26:596–605.
16 Murray PE, Smith AJ, Garcia-Godoy F, Lumley PJ. Comparison of operative procedure variables on pulpal viability in an ex vivo model. Int Endod J 2008;41:389–400.
17 Leksell E, Ridell K, Cvek M, Mejàre I: Pulpal exposure after stepwise versus direct complete excavation of deep carious lesions in young posterior permanent teeth. Endod Dent Traumatol 1996;12: 192–196.
18 Magnusson BO, Sundell SO: Stepwise excavation of deep carious lesions in primary molars. J Int Assoc Dent Child 1977;8:36–40.
19 Barthel CR, Rosenkranz B, Leuenberg A, Roulet JF: Pulp capping of carious exposures: treatment outcome after 5 and 10 years: a retrospective study. J Endod 2000;26:525–528.
20 Bogen G, Kim JS, Bakland LK: Direct pulp capping with mineral trioxide aggregate: an observational study. J Am Dent Assoc 2008;139:305–315.
21 Hatton JF, Pashley DH, Shunk J, Stewart GP: In vitro and in vivo measurement of remaining dentin thickness. J Endod 1994;20:580–584.
22 Yoshida H, Tsuji M, Matsumoto H: An electrical method for examining remaining dentine thickness. J Dent 1989;17:284–286.
23 Teilmans S, Bergmans L, Duvck J, Naert I: Evaluation of a preparation depth controlling device: a pilot study. Quintessence Int 2007;38:135–142.
24 Hume WR: Need for change in standards of caries diagnosis – perspective based on the structure and behaviour of the caries lesion. J Dent Educ 1993; 57:439–443.
25 Handelman SL, Washburn F, Wopperer P: Two year report of sealant effect on bacteria in dental caries. J Am Dent Assoc 1976;93:967–970.
26 Mertz-Fairhurst EJ, Schuster GS, Williams JE, Fairhurst CW: Clinical progress of sealed and unsealed caries. I. Depth changes and bacterial counts. J Prosthet Dent 1979;42:521–526.
27 Mertz-Fairhurst EJ, Schuster GS, Williams JE, Fairhurst CW: Clinical progress of sealed and unsealed caries. II. Standardized radiographs and clinical observation. J Prosthet Dent 1979;42:633–637.
28 Jensen OE, Handelman SL: Effect of an autopolymerising sealant on viability of microflora in occlusal dental caries. Scand J Dent Res 1980;88:382–388.
29 Handelman SL, Leverett DH, Espeland MA, Curzon JA: Clinical radiographic evaluation of sealed carious and sound tooth surfaces. J Am Dent Assoc 1986;113:751–754.
30 Handelman SL, Leverett DH, Espeland MA, Curzon JA: Retention of sealants over carious and sound surfaces. Community Dent Oral Epidemiol 1987;15: 1–5.
31 Ahovuo-Saloranta A, Hiiri A, Nordblad A, Mäkelä M, Worthington HV: Pit and fissure sealants for preventing dental decay in permanent teeth of children and adolescents. Cochrane Database Syst Rev 2008;8:CD001830.
32 Mertz-Fairhurst EJ, Curtis JW Jr, Ergle JW, Rueggeberg FA, Adair SM: Ultraconservative and cariostatic sealed restorations: results at year 10. J Am Dent Assoc 1998;129:55–66.

33 Mertz-Fairhurst EJ, Call-Smith KM, Shuster GS, Williams JE, Davis QB, Smith CD, Bell RA, Sherrer JD, Myers DR, Morse PK, et al: Clinical performance of sealed composite restorations placed over caries compared with sealed and unsealed amalgam restorations. J Am Dent Assoc 1987;115:689–694.

34 Mertz-Fairhurst EJ, Williams JE, Schuster GS, Smith CD, Pierce KL, Mackert JR Jr, Sherrer JD, Wenner KK, Davis QB, Garman TA, et al: Ultraconservative sealed restorations: three year results. J Public Health Dent 1991;51:239–250.

35 Mertz-Fairhurst EJ, Williams JE, Pierce KL, Smith CD, Schuster GS, Mackert JR Jr, Sherrer JD, Wenner KK, Richards EE, Davis QB, et al: Sealed restorations: 4-year results. Am J Dent 1991;4:43–49.

36 Mertz-Fairhurst EJ, Richards EE, Williams JE, Smith CD, Mackert JR Jr, Schuster GS, Sherrer JD, O'Dell NL, Pierce KL, Wenner KK, et al: Sealed restorations: 5-year results. Am J Dent 1992;5:5–10.

37 Mertz-Fairhurst EJ, Smith CD, Williams JE, Sherrer JD, Mackert JR Jr, Richards EE, Schuster GS, O'Dell NL, Pierce KL, Kovarik RE, et al: Cariostatic and ultraconservative sealed restorations: six-year results. Quintessence Int 1992;23:827–838.

38 Mertz-Fairhurst EJ, Adair SM, Sams DR, Curtis JW Jr, Ergle JW, Hawkins KI, Mackert JR Jr, O'Dell NL, Richards EE, Rueggeberg F, et al: Cariostatic and ultraconservative sealed restorations: nine-year results among children and adults. ASDC J Dent Child 1995;62:97–107.

39 Bjørndal L, Larsen T, Thylstrup A: A clinical and microbiological study of deep carious lesions during stepwise excavation using long treatment intervals. Caries Res 1997;31:411–417.

40 Bjørndal L, Thylstrup A: A practice-based study on stepwise excavation of deep carious lesions in permanent teeth: a 1 year follow-up study. Community Dent Oral Epidemiol 1998;26:122–128.

41 Maltz M, Oliveira EF, Fontanella V, Carminatti G: Deep caries lesions after incomplete dentine caries removal: 40 month follow-up study. Caries Res 2007;41:493–496.

42 Paddick JS, Brailsford SR, Kidd EA, Beighton D: Phenotypic and genotypic selection of microbiota surviving under dental restorations. Appl Environ Microbiol 2005;71:2467–2472.

43 Ricketts DN, Kidd EA, Innes N, Clarkson J: Complete or ultraconservative removal of decayed tissue in unfilled teeth. Cochrane Database Syst Rev 2006; 3:CD003808.

44 Ribeiro CCC, Baratieri LN, Perdigao J, Baratieri NMM, Ritter AV: A clinical, radiographic, and scanning electron microscopic evaluation of adhesive restorations on carious dentin in primary teeth. Quintessence Int 1999;30:591–599.

45 Maltz M, de Oliveira EF, Fontanella V, Bianchi R: A clinical and radiographic study of deep caries lesions after incomplete caries removal. Quintessence Int 2002;33:151–159.

46 Bjørndal L: Indirect pulp therapy and stepwise excavation. Pediatr Dent 2008;30:225–229.

47 Innes NP, Stirrups DR, Evans DJ, Hall N, Leggate M: A novel technique using preformed metal crowns for managing carious primary molars in general practice – a retrospective analysis. Br Dent J 2006; 200:451–454.

48 Innes NPT, Evans DJP, Stirrups DR: The Hall technique: a randomized controlled clinical trial of a novel method of managing carious primary molars in general dental practice: acceptability of the technique and outcomes at 23 months. BMC Oral Health 2007;7:18.

49 Martignon S, Ekstrand KR, Ellwood R: Efficacy of sealing proximal early active lesions: an 18-month clinical study evaluated by conventional and subtraction radiography. Caries Res 2006;40:382–388.

50 Ricketts DN, Ekstrand KR, Martignon S, Ellwood R, Alatsaris M, Nugent Z: Accuracy and reproducibility of conventional radiographic assessment and subtraction radiography in detecting demineralization in occlusal surfaces. Caries Res 2007;41:121–128.

David Ricketts
Dundee Dental Hospital and School
Park Place
Dundee DD1 4HR (UK)
Tel./Fax +44 1382 635984, E-Mail d.n.j.ricketts@dundee.ac.uk

Recall, Reassessment and Monitoring

J.E. Clarkson[a] · B.T. Amaechi[b] · H. Ngo[c] · D. Bonetti[a]

[a]Dental Health Services and Research Unit, University of Dundee, Dundee, UK; [b]Department of Community Dentistry, UTHSCSA, San Antonio, Tex. USA; [c]Department of Otolaryngology – Head & Neck Surgery, National University Hospital, Singapore

Abstract

A recall system is a continuing care regime which provides opportunities to reassess and monitor the oral health of patients and to inform future treatment planning. There is some evidence that recall visits have a positive impact on the natural and functional dentition. Unfortunately, there is a general paucity of reliable evidence about the timing of recall visits despite the widely adopted 6-month interval. In response to political, professional and patient uncertainty, the UK National Institute of Health and Clinical Excellence (NICE) convened a guideline development group to consider both best evidence and best practice in this field. The NICE issued a guidance document in 2004 recommending that the individual risk status should determine the patient's recall interval. The recommendations cover risk factors such as caries incidence and restorations; periodontal health and tooth loss, patients' well-being, general health and preventive habits, pain and anxiety. Methods and tools to facilitate and standardize the collection of risk information are currently being developed and/or collated by the Scottish Dental Clinical Effectiveness Programme. The selection of a recall interval is a multifaceted and complex decision involving the judgement of both clinician and patient. More research is needed into the rate of progression of oral diseases and the impact of recall on oral health and quality of life. Nevertheless, the NICE guidance is based on the best available evidence, and it should be used to determine personalized variable time intervals to assess, reassess and monitor the oral health and caries status of patients.

Copyright © 2009 S. Karger AG, Basel

A recall system is a means of establishing a continuing care regime. It provides opportunities to reassess and monitor the oral health of patients. This is increasingly related to disease prevention, the early detection of any newly developed disease (in order to deliver prompt preventive care) or determining the status of a previously diagnosed and treated disease. Reassessing and monitoring during a treatment period will also enable the clinician or the patient to consider altering the treatment regimen to obtain a more favourable outcome. Furthermore, having the opportunity to determine the effectiveness of previous treatment and treatment decisions may provide evidence for future clinical governance and quality improvement services. Additionally, recall visits provide opportunities to provide advice, reassess and reinforce the appropriateness of previous advice, monitor patient compliance with previous advice and treatment, as well as to encourage patient behaviour that will improve and maintain their oral and general health.

There is some evidence that recall visits, irrespective of the frequency, have a positive impact in terms of the comparative preservation of the natural and functional dentition. For example, a systematic review found 12 studies which reported an increase in decay with a decrease in dental check frequency (8 of which were significant differences) and 6 studies which reported a decrease in filled teeth/surfaces with a decrease in dental check frequency [1]. Boehmer et al. [2] reported fewer decayed coronal surfaces and significantly fewer untreated root caries lesions in patients that had attended a dentist during the previous 2 years than in patients who had attended 2 or more years before. Thomson [3] reported that problem-oriented attenders had significantly higher DMFS and DFS increment scores compared with patients who attended for check-ups. Bullock et al. [4] compared regular attenders with casual attenders and found a significant increase in the proportion of subjects with visual caries causing cavitation with a decrease in dental check frequency. The same study reported a significant increase in the proportion of subjects with dentinal caries on bitewing radiographs with a decrease in dental check frequency. These differences persisted after adjusting for age, gender, social class and smoking. Freire et al. [5] reported an increased risk of having a high caries severity among those who attended the dentists mainly when in trouble, compared with those attending mainly for check-ups.

Unfortunately, reviews and systematic reviews have also underpinned the general paucity of reliable scientific evidence in relation to this area of dental practice [1, 6–9]. The available evidence in relation to many aspects of dental recall intervals is weak and conflicting, and there is a lack of high-quality research to properly inform clinical practice on the timing of recall visits. Nevertheless, a 6-month interval between recall appointments has been widely adopted as an aim around the world by both patients and clinicians. In fact, in many cases, the actual interval between typical recall appointments greatly exceeds this target. Some health organizations, including the National Health Service (NHS) in the UK, have implicitly recognized this interval by remunerating dental practitioners for patients' 6-monthly check-ups. The evolution of this sacrosanct view is anecdotally reported to have been popularized initially by dentifrice advertising in the late 40s.

The growing realization that this might not be the best basis to determine oral health resource management has generated significant international debate over the appropriate timing of recall intervals for dental check-ups. A number of political and professional issues have fuelled this debate. Foremost is the scarcity of supporting evidence for the timing of recall intervals, particularly for the commonly accepted 6-monthly recall [10]. For example, the Health Technology Assessment systematic review of routine dental checks found little evidence to support or refute the practice of encouraging the 6-monthly traditional dental checks in adults. Additionally, the more recent Cochrane review also concluded that there was insufficient evidence to support the potential beneficial or harmful effects of the 6-monthly recall interval between dental check-ups on patient outcomes, provider workload and health care costs [10]. Other issues generating the recall interval debate are the international paradigm shift from treatment- to patient-centred services, the evolution of caries management from its previous repair and restoration focus to one of conservation and prevention, as well as the recent development and introduction of the International Caries Detection and Assessment System [11–13] which allows classification and recording of the early stages of caries which are amenable to preventive treatment options.

The UK Experience

A recall system of '6-monthly' dental check-ups has been customary in the General Dental Service in the UK since the inception of the NHS. In keeping with the international impetus toward patient-centred services, the Department of Health issued a strategy document 'Modernising NHS dentistry – implementing the NHS plan'. The government explicitly stated its intention to examine the evidence for changing working practices 'including more flexible recall intervals for routine examinations, to ensure the most appropriate treatment and care for patients' [14]. It was argued that patients should be recalled at intervals matching their individual needs rather than a generalized service requirement [14]. This view was reiterated in the assessment of primary care dental services by the audit commission, which suggested that evidence-based criteria should be introduced to determine the best check-up attendance interval for each individual patient [15].

Furthermore, the UK government's increasing awareness that oral health is an important component of general health, combined with its desire to improve general well-being of patients and patient safety, generated the production of the Department of Health's strategy document 'NHS dentistry: options for change in 2002' and the subsequent legislation to change the organization of dental services and the way in which oral health is assessed [16]. This document was informed by the body of evidence showing that caries is the most prevalent infectious disease of both children and adults, that it occurs on a continuous scale from subclinical lesions to tissue damage leading to pulpal exposure, and that there are wide variations between patients in their susceptibility to this disease, the likelihood of early disease progression and the speed of disease progression if it occurs. It was concluded that a blanket 6-monthly recall policy is just too rigid to take into account these individual need differences. The document recommended that a standardized comprehensive oral health assessment should involve taking full histories, a thorough dental, head and neck examination, the provision of preventive advice and a personalized care plan to be determined by both dentist and patient, including when the next oral health review is to take place.

In response to this NHS pressure, as well as to professional and patient uncertainty, the National Institute of Health and Clinical Excellence (NICE) issued a guidance document in 2004 recommending that the individual patient's caries risk status should inform his/her recall interval [17]. The guideline recommendations were based on the best available evidence from reviews of published guidelines from different health authorities and professional organizations, including the Health Technology Assessment [1], Department of Health [14], the American Academy of Pediatric Dentistry [18], systematic reviews and other research evidence relating to risk factors for oral disease and on the effectiveness of dental health education and oral health promotion [17]. The guideline looked at the potential of both the patient and the dental team to improve or maintain the patient's quality of life and to reduce morbidity associated with oral and dental disease. The guidance indicates that the recall interval range should vary from 3 to 24 months, according to risk (that is 3–12 months for children of less than 18 years and 3–24 months for adults of 18 or more years).The recommendations covered a broad array of possible risk factors for which there was evidence, including caries incidence and restorations, periodontal health and tooth loss, as well as the patients' well-being, general health and preventive habits, pain and anxiety. According to the levels of evidence used by the Scottish Dental Clinical Effectiveness Programme (SDCEP), most of the recommendations made by the NICE were graded as R_e (recommendation based on consensus of expert opinion) or R_w (recommendation supported by weak evidence with some potential for bias).

The key NICE guideline recommendations are to:
- *personalize* recall intervals based on an assessment of each patient's disease levels and risk of or from dental disease;
- *integrate* this assessment with the guideline evidence, the clinical judgement and expertise of the dental team, and discussions with the patient; *ensure* that comprehensive histories are taken, examinations are conducted and initial preventive advice is given; this will allow the dental team and the patient (and/or his or her parent, guardian or carer) to discuss, where appropriate:
  - the effects of oral hygiene, diet, fluoride use, tobacco and alcohol on oral health (R_s, recommendation supported by strong evidence with limited bias);
  - the risk factors that may influence the patient's oral health and their implications for deciding the appropriate recall interval;
  - the outcome of previous care episodes and the suitability of previously recommended intervals;
  - the patient's ability or desire to visit the dentist at the recommended interval (R_e);
  - the financial costs to the patient of having the oral health review and any subsequent treatments;
- *choose* the recall interval either at the end of an oral health review if no further treatment is indicated, or on completion of a specific treatment journey; the recommended shortest and longest intervals between oral health reviews are as follows:

- the shortest interval between oral health reviews for all patients should be 3 months;
- the longest interval between oral health reviews for patients younger than 18 years should be 12 months;
- the longest interval between oral health reviews for patients aged 18 years and older should be 24 months:

'There is evidence that the rate of progression of dental caries can be more rapid in children and adolescents than in older people, and it seems to be faster in primary teeth than in permanent teeth (see full guideline). Periodic developmental assessment of the dentition is also required in children. Recall intervals of no longer than 12 months give the opportunity for delivering and reinforcing preventive advice and for raising awareness of the importance of good oral health. This is particularly important in young children, to lay the foundations for life-long dental health.'

- *assign* a recall interval of 3, 6, 9 or 12 months if a patient is younger than 18 years, or 3, 6, 9, 12, 15, 18, 21 or 24 months if he or she is aged 18 years or older:

'The interval may be maintained at the same level if it is achieving its aims. For someone with low disease activity, it may be possible to gradually extend the interval towards the 24-month maximum period – once the patient and the dental team are confident that this is satisfactory. Patients whose disease activity continues unabated may need a shorter interval and may need more intensive preventive care and closer supervision. Patients should be encouraged to seek advice from a dentist before their next scheduled review if there are any significant changes in their risk factors. They also need to understand that (as is the case with the current 6-month recall regimen) there is no guarantee that new disease will not develop between recall visits.'

- *discuss* the recommended recall interval with the patient and record this interval, and the patient's agreement or disagreement with it, in the current record-keeping system;
- *review* the recall interval at the next oral health review, in order to learn from the patient's responses to the oral care provided and the health outcomes achieved; this feedback and the findings of the oral health review should be used to adjust the next recall interval chosen;
- *inform* patients that their recommended recall interval may vary over time; it is important to engage the patients in the treatment of caries because a high level of compliance is required for its success; it also follows that monitoring and recall are essential in the management of caries.

Figure 1 presents an overview of the evidence-based procedure for determining the recall interval between routine dental examinations. Figure 2 is the NICE dental recall checklist of modifying factors of caries risk, which was developed to assist the evaluation and prediction of risk. The checklist includes age, medical history, social history, dietary habits, exposure to fluoride, clinical evidence and dental history, recent and previous caries experience, recent and previous periodontal disease experience, mucosal lesions, plaque, saliva flow rate, erosion and tooth surface loss.

However, assessing the risk of developing oral disease is not a perfect science. Methods and tools to help standardize and facilitate the collection of the risk and protective factor information identified by the NICE guideline are currently being developed and collated under the SDCEP [19]. Once piloted and finalized, these methods and tools will be presented in a SDCEP supplementary guidance document on how to pull together the relevant information to form diagnoses, to identify the level of individual patient risk for the development and/or progression of oral disease and to enable the development of a care plan, which includes a personalized recall interval appropriate for that patient's risk status at that point in time.

One of these tools is the International Caries Detection and Assessment System [11–13]. Currently, UK dentists use a variety of charting systems to highlight the patient's clinical caries status before treatment, although a baseline standardized charting system with International Dental Federation tooth numbering is recommended. However, most recording systems currently in use do not readily enable the accurate recording of the various stages in the caries process (from first visual enamel surface change to an extensive cavity). Increasing the accuracy of risk assessment requires the need for a more detailed approach to recording and monitoring the caries process. The International Caries Detection and Assessment System is a clinical visual scoring system that is based on international best evidence and is designed for use in dental clinical practice, as well as in education, clinical research and epidemiology. This scale enables the collation of high-quality information on caries status to help inform decisions about appropriate diagnosis and prognosis at the individual patient level. Using this tool at each recall visit would enable the reassessment and monitoring essential to the identification of personalized preventive and operative care needs that should be behind the determination of the next recall visit.

Nevertheless, even with the NICE recommendations and the development and collation of standardized tools and methods by the SDCEP to facilitate the implementation of those recommendations, the process of appropriate setting of recall still has a long way to go. Uncertainty remains among dentists as to how best to implement the guidance in practice. The selection of an appropriate recall interval for a patient is a multifaceted decision that involves the judgement of both clinician and patient and cannot be decided in a completely mechanistic fashion, whatever tools are produced – particularly when those tools are not comprehensive. The NICE checklist information is not an exhaustive list of factors that may influence the choice of a recall interval for a patient [8]. For example, the presence of implants or fixed and removable prostheses is not mentioned as a risk factor for caries, periodontal or mucosal disease. Likewise, specific risk periods for caries, such as the eruption of second molars, are not discussed [8]. Furthermore, there is insufficient evidence to assign a 'weight' to individual factors that are in the checklist, and dentists must use their clinical judgement to weigh the risk and protective factors for each patient.

Additionally, it is to be remembered that many of the NICE recommendations determining the length of recall intervals were based on the clinical experience of the Guideline Development Group and advice received during the consultation process. The lack of scientific evidence behind differing recall strategies complicates the adoption process. While it is anticipated that carrying out a comprehensive history

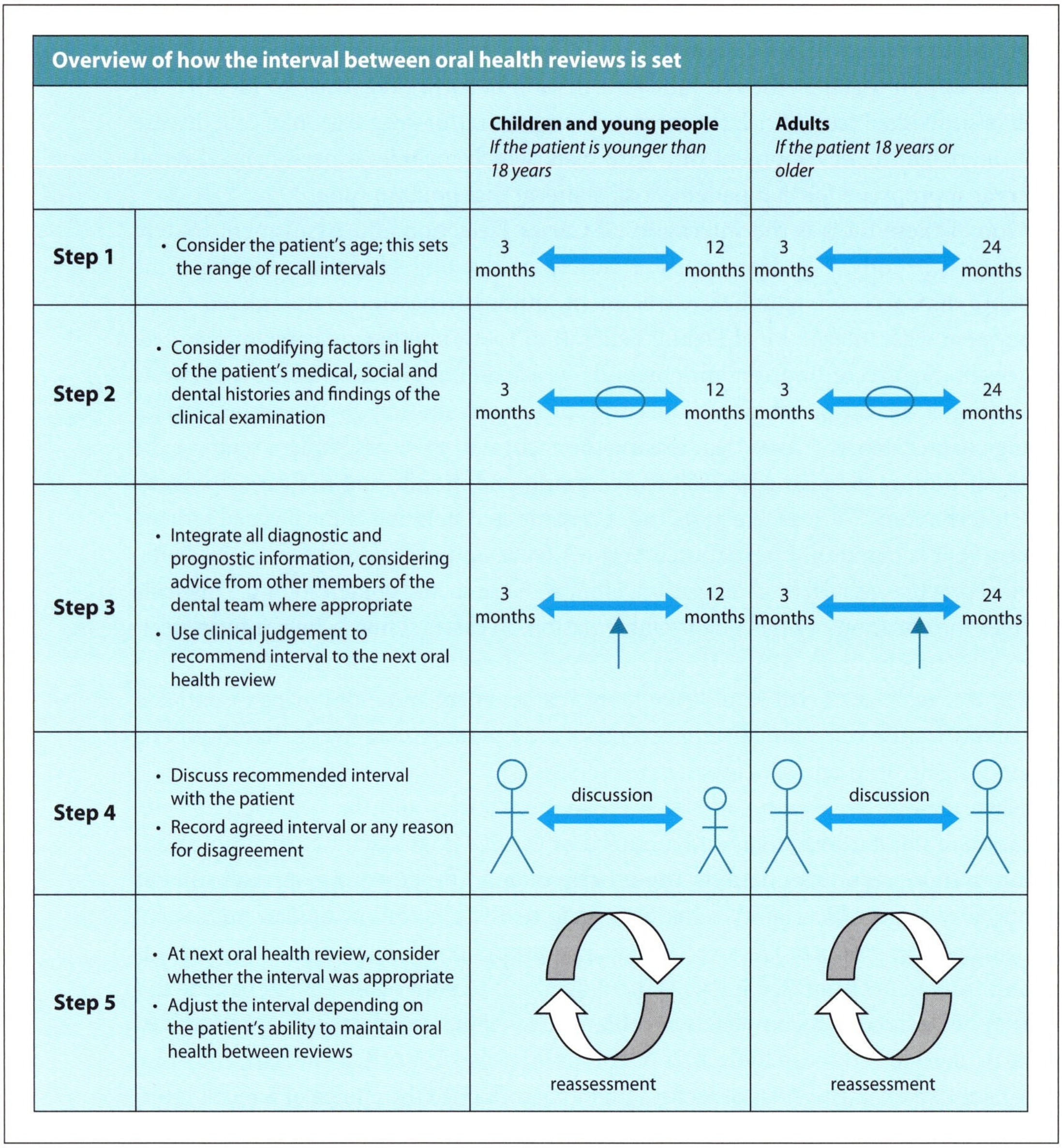

		Children and young people If the patient is younger than 18 years	Adults If the patient 18 years or older
Step 1	• Consider the patient's age; this sets the range of recall intervals	3 months ↔ 12 months	3 months ↔ 24 months
Step 2	• Consider modifying factors in light of the patient's medical, social and dental histories and findings of the clinical examination	3 months ↔ 12 months	3 months ↔ 24 months
Step 3	• Integrate all diagnostic and prognostic information, considering advice from other members of the dental team where appropriate • Use clinical judgement to recommend interval to the next oral health review	3 months ↔ 12 months	3 months ↔ 24 months
Step 4	• Discuss recommended interval with the patient • Record agreed interval or any reason for disagreement	discussion	discussion
Step 5	• At next oral health review, consider whether the interval was appropriate • Adjust the interval depending on the patient's ability to maintain oral health between reviews	reassessment	reassessment

Fig. 1. An overview of the recommended method of determining a personalized recall interval (NICE guideline on dental recall [17]).

Fig. 2. Checklist of modifying factors for risk assessment (NICE guideline on dental recall [17]). BPE = Basic periodontal examination.

Checklist of modifying factors

Name: _____ Date of birth: _____

	Oral health review date:			
		Yes No	Yes No	Yes No
Medical history				
Conditions where dental disease could put the patient's general health at increased risk (such as cardiovascular disease, bleeding disorders, immunosuppression)		☐ ☐	☐ ☐	☐ ☐
Conditions that increase a patient's risk of developing dental disease (such as diabetes, xerostomia)		☐ ☐	☐ ☐	☐ ☐
Conditions that may complicate dental treatment or the patient's ability to maintain their oral health (such as special needs, anxious/nervous/phobic conditions)		☐ ☐	☐ ☐	☐ ☐
Social history				
High caries in mother and siblings		☐ ☐	☐ ☐	☐ ☐
Tobacco use		☐ ☐	☐ ☐	☐ ☐
Excessive alcohol use		☐ ☐	☐ ☐	☐ ☐
Family history of chronic or aggressive (early onset/juvenile) periodontitis		☐ ☐	☐ ☐	☐ ☐
Dietary habits				
High and/or frequent sugar intake		☐ ☐	☐ ☐	☐ ☐
High and/or frequent dietary acid intake		☐ ☐	☐ ☐	☐ ☐
Exposure to fluoride				
Use of fluoride toothpast		☐ ☐	☐ ☐	☐ ☐
other sources of fluoride (for example, the patients live in a water-fluoridated area)		☐ ☐	☐ ☐	☐ ☐
Clinical evidence and dental history				
Recent and previous caries experience				
New lesions since last check-up		☐ ☐	☐ ☐	☐ ☐
Anterior caries or restorations		☐ ☐	☐ ☐	☐ ☐
Premature extractions because of caries		☐ ☐	☐ ☐	☐ ☐
Past root caries or large number of exposed roots		☐ ☐	☐ ☐	☐ ☐
Heavily restored dentition		☐ ☐	☐ ☐	☐ ☐
Recent and previous periodontal disease experience				
Previous history of periodontal disease		☐ ☐	☐ ☐	☐ ☐
Evidence of gingivitis		☐ ☐	☐ ☐	☐ ☐
Presence of periodontal pockets (BPE code 3 or 4) and/or bleeding on probing		☐ ☐	☐ ☐	☐ ☐
Presence of furcation involvement or advanced attachment loss (BPE code*)		☐ ☐	☐ ☐	☐ ☐
Mucosal lesions				
Muscosal lesion present		☐ ☐	☐ ☐	☐ ☐
Plaque				
Poor level of oral hygiene		☐ ☐	☐ ☐	☐ ☐
Plaque-retaining facotrs (such as orthodontic appliances)		☐ ☐	☐ ☐	☐ ☐
Saliva				
Low saliva flow rate		☐ ☐	☐ ☐	☐ ☐
Erosion and tooth surface loss				
Clinical evidence of tooth wear		☐ ☐	☐ ☐	☐ ☐
Recommended recall interval for next oral health review:		Months	Months	Months
Does patient agree with recommended interval? If 'No', record reason for disagreement in notes		Yes No	Yes No	Yes No

BPE code* is used when attachment loss is ≥7 mm and/or furcation involvements are present and extended dental examination will better inform the dentist as to the patient's care needs, there remains little evidence how this actually relates to the oral health, quality of life and dental anxiety of the patients [17]. It may therefore prove difficult to wean clinicians from their current behaviour of setting 6-monthly recalls, since this approach does not entail coping with the clinical examinations and paperwork required to determine a personalized recall interval within the constraints of a primary care consultation. Effective communication, practising within medicolegal constraints and comprehensive and accurate record keeping are also variables that may influence the NICE recommended process of setting risk-adjusted recall intervals in the primary care environment.

Furthermore, while there is a body of opinion that believes extending the interval between check-up appointments increases the opportunity for access to dental services and reduces patients' exposure to the risks of unnecessary interventions, other factors may be more important to dentists and patients. Anecdotal evidence from interviews conducted by the authors was that dentists were anxious that their patients would perceive a recall interval longer than 6 months as a breach of a professional duty of care. This may be indicative that recall strategies other than the long accepted period of 6 months are likely to vary in terms of non-health outcomes which are not taken into account in the NICE recall interval determination process. A series of in-depth interviews were recently conducted with adults in Scotland and Southern England investigating service users' feelings and opinions of the recall visit. In line with the results of other studies, users commented that the 6-monthly dental recall visit provided: reassurance – 'I feel quite secure that there's nothing going too wrong' – as well as increased confidence in their oral health – 'it just gives you a sense of confidence, self-confidence and well-being' [20, 21].

There is little question that further research is needed to:
1 assess the relative effectiveness of different recall intervals for dental check-ups for different caries risk status;
2 develop and validate efficient, cost- and time-effective tools to facilitate risk-based assessment of an individual patient's dental history and oral health status, e.g. chair side devices, electronic tools;
3 examine the impact of recall, reassessment and monitoring on oral health and quality of life of the patient;
4 determine the rate of progression of oral diseases;
5 compare the outcomes of providing advice and preventive measures against oral diseases;
6 examine the impact of recall intervals on patient views and expectations of their dentist and dental treatment;
7 examine the effects on periodontal health of routine scale and polish treatment (in conjunction with oral hygiene instruction) in different populations; specifically, research is needed to examine the clinical effectiveness and cost-effectiveness of providing this intervention at different time intervals;

8 determine how often each risk factor should be reviewed and how (e.g. bitewing radiograph, saliva assessment);
9 validate the current assumed predictors of future caries development in children and adults.

Some of these issues are currently being addressed. The Dental Health Services Research Unit in Scotland, SDCEP and the Universities of Dundee, Aberdeen, Edinburgh and Newcastle, as well as Scottish and English Primary Care Research Networks are in the initial processes of conducting a trial to investigate whether fixed-period 24-month or risk-based recall intervals are more effective and cost-effective in maintaining oral health than the traditional fixed-period 6-month recall. The secondary objectives of the trial are to compare the effect of different recall intervals on the provision and use of dental services (process of care including preventive and interventive care), on patients' anxiety, satisfaction with care, oral health knowledge, attitudes and behaviours, as well as on their economic costs and benefits. The impact of dentists' professional engagement, work-related stress and psychological health will also be explored.

Conclusion

Patient-centred comprehensive caries management will require the implementation of a new approach to determine the recall interval for most patients. While more research is needed and a support infrastructure should be developed to enhance and enable the judgement of both clinician and patient in the care process, the NICE guideline is based on the best available evidence, and the authors of this chapter recommend using it to determine personalized variable time intervals to assess, reassess and monitor the oral health of patients.

References

1 Davenport C, Elley K, Salas C, Taylor-Weetman CL, Fry-Smith A, Bryan S, et al: The clinical effectiveness and cost-effectiveness of routine dental checks: a systematic review and economic evaluation. Health Technol Assess 2003;7:iii–127.
2 Boehmer U, Kressin NR, Spiro A III, et al: Oral health of ambulatory care patients. Mil Med 2001; 166:171–178.
3 Thomson WM: Use of dental services by 26-year-old New Zealanders. NZ Dent J 2001;97:44–48.
4 Bullock C, Boath E, Lewis M, et al: A case control study of differences between regular and casual adult attenders in general dental practice. Prim Dent Care 2001;8:35–40.
5 Freire M, Hardy R, Sheiham A: Mothers' sense of coherence and their adolescent children's oral health status and behaviours. Community Dent Health 2002;19:24–31.
6 Bader JD, Shugars DA, Bonito AJ: A systematic review of selected caries prevention and management methods. Community Dent Oral Epidemiol 2001;29:399–411.
7 Bader J, et al: Diagnosis and management of dental caries throughout life. J Dent Educ 2002;65:1162–1168.
8 Bader J: Risk-based recall intervals recommended. Evid Based Dent 2005;6:2–4.

9 Beirne P, Forgie A, Clarkson JE, Worthington HV: Recall intervals for oral health in primary care patients. Aust Dent J 2005;50:209–210.
10 Beirne P, Forgie A, Worthington HV, Clarkson JE: Routine scale and polish for periodontal health in adults. Cochrane Database Syst Rev 2005;1: CD004625.
11 Ismail AI, Sohn W, Tellez M, Amaya A, Sen A, Hasson H, et al: The International Caries Detection and Assessment System (ICDAS): an integrated system for measuring dental caries. Community Dent Oral Epidemiol 2007;35:170–178.
12 ICDAS Coordinating Committee: International Caries Detection and Assessment System (ICDAS): rationale and evidence for the International Caries Detection and Assessment System (ICDAS II); in Stookey GK (ed): Clinical Models Workshop: Remin-Demin, Precavitation, Caries – proceedings of the 7th Indiana Conference. Indianapolis, Indiana University School of Dentistry, 2005, pp 161–221.
13 Chesters RK, Pitts NB, Matuliene G, Kvedariene A, Huntington E, Bendinskaite R, et al: An abbreviated caries clinical trial design validated over 24 months. J Dent Res 2002;81:637–640.
14 Department of Health: Modernizing NHS dentistry: implementing the NHS plan. London, Department of Health, 2000.
15 Audit Commission: Dentistry: primary dental care services in England and Wales. London, Audit Commission, 2000.
16 Department of Health: NHS dentistry: options for change. London, Department of Health, 2000.
17 National Institute for Clinical Excellence (NICE): Guide on dental recall: recall interval between routine dental examinations. Clinical guideline 19. London, October 2004. www.nice.org.uk/CG019 NICEguideline (accessed March 2009).
18 American Academy of Pediatric Dentistry: Clinical guideline on periodicity of examination, preventive dental services, anticipatory guidance and oral treatment for children. 2003. http://www.aapd.org (accessed March 2009).
19 Scottish Dental Clinical Effectiveness Programme. Oral Health Assessment. NHS Education Scotland 2006. February 5, 2007.
20 Gibson BJ, Drennan J, Hanna S, Freeman R: An exploratory qualitative study examining the social and psychological processes involved in regular dental attendance. J Public Health Dent 2000;60:5–11.
21 Wyrwich KW, Tardino VM: Understanding global transition assessments. Qual Life Res 2006;15:995–1004.

J.E. Clarkson
Dental Health Services and Research Unit, University of Dundee
Mackenzie Building, Kirsty Semple Way
Dundee DD2 4BF (UK)
Tel. +44 1382 420060, Fax +44 1382 420051, E-Mail j.e.clarkson@cpse.dundee.ac.uk

Implementation

Improving Caries Detection, Assessment, Diagnosis and Monitoring

N.B. Pitts

Dental Health Services and Research Unit, University of Dundee, Dundee, UK

Abstract

This chapter deals with improving the detection, assessment, diagnosis and monitoring of caries to ensure optimal *personalized caries management*. This can be achieved by delivering what we have (synthesized evidence and international consensus) better and more consistently, as well as driving research and innovation in the areas where we need them. There is a need to better understand the interrelated pieces of the jigsaw that makes up evidence-based dentistry, i.e. the linkages between (a) research and synthesis, (b) dissemination of research results and (c) the implementation of research findings which should ensure that research findings change practice at the clinician-patient level. The *current situation* is outlined; it is at the implementation step where preventive caries control seems to have failed in some countries but not others. *Opportunities for implementation* include: capitalizing on the World Health Organization's global policy for improvement of oral health, which sets out an action plan for health promotion and *integrated disease prevention*; utilizing the developments around the International Caries Detection and Assessment System wardrobe of options and e-learning; building on initiatives from the International Dental Federation and the American Dental Association and linking these to patients' preferences, the wider moves to wellbeing and health maintenance. *Challenges for implementation* include the slow pace of evolution around dental remuneration systems and some groups of dentists failing to embrace clinical prevention. In the future, implementation of current and developing evidence should be accompanied by research into getting research findings into routine practice, with impacts on the behaviour of patients, professionals and policy makers.

Copyright © 2009 S. Karger AG, Basel

This chapter deals with improving the detection, assessment, diagnosis and monitoring of caries to ensure optimal *personalized caries management* including clinical prevention and caries control. This can be achieved by delivering what we have (synthesized evidence and international consensus) better and more consistently, as well as driving research and innovation in the areas where we need them.

The details of much of what we have and the areas in which we need more high-quality research have been outlined in the preceding chapters of this book. The focus of this chapter is more specifically around the implementation of research findings in these areas of clinical cariology. The discussion will cover the present situation, the opportunities and the challenges to implementation of research findings in the area and will also provide the start of a map to the future

Evidence-Based Dentistry and the Collaboration for Improving Dentistry

The chapter by Pitts [this vol., pp. 1–14] provides an overview of the background issues, including the continuing burden of preventable disease that dental caries represents on a global scale and the development of tools to provide a sound foundation of lesion detection, assessment and diagnosis which, when combined with appropriate patient level risk information and monitoring, enables effective treatment planning. The International Caries Detection and Assessment System (ICDAS), building on cariology research from over 50 years, which can enable this process [1], was also outlined. Despite this progress and evidence that a purely restorative approach will not 'cure' the disease, preventive caries control has been slow to be adopted in many countries, but not others [2].

The concepts of evidence-based dentistry were also outlined in the same chapter. There is a need to understand in more depth the interrelated pieces of the jigsaw that makes up evidence-based dentistry. There are ideally meant to be smooth linkages between (a) research and synthesis [3], (b) dissemination of research results [4] and (c) the implementation of research findings [5]. However, in practice, in dentistry as in many other fields of health care, these linkages are often slow and unpredictable.

Figure 1 outlines a triangular representation of what should be a continuing cycle to get evidence into practice; it is called the Collaboration for Improving Dentistry model.

The dynamic linkages between these elements, along the sides of the triangle as well as linking between the 3 arms, are all vital to moving evidence-based dentistry forward. Although it can prove hard to achieve, following this process and ensuring wider communication between the various stakeholders should ensure that:
- an informed research agenda adds to the systematically updated evidence base;
- the findings of research are disseminated actively, and
- implementation of the findings can change practice at the clinician-patient level.

Implementation research, and indeed implementation science, is a relatively new activity but is seen as increasingly important in the developing field of 'translational medicine'. The focus is not just at the initial linkages between laboratory bench and patient bedside in a hospital research setting (so-called type 1 translational medicine), but also broader to include a wider use of innovations at the patient (type 2) and community/policy levels (type 3). The need to make more consistent progress in translating cariology research into routine clinical care planning and practice is to look at how best to deliver the full translational medicine continuum, that is from bench → chairside → individual patient → populations → policy makers and back again.

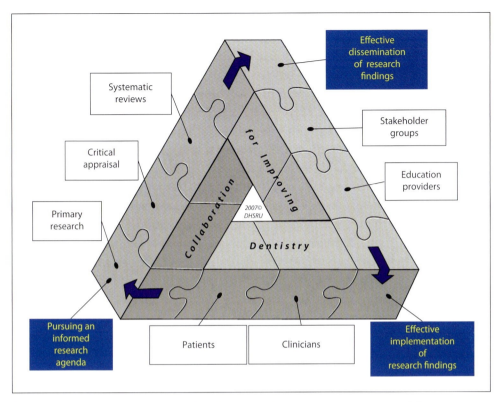

Fig. 1. Triangular representation of the Collaboration for Improving Dentistry model.

This work has started to be reported in dentistry, for example by applying psychological theory to evidence-based practice in seeking to identify factors predictive of taking intra-oral radiographs [6]. The results of this investigation suggest that an intervention targeting predictive psychological variables could increase the implementation of evidence-based practice, while simply influencing knowledge is unlikely to do so. The field is complex and truly multidisciplinary.

While the so-called hierarchy of evidence relating to randomized controlled trials continues to play an important role in understanding clinical interventions and producing guidance, there is a growing awareness of the need to also integrate qualitative evidence and a consensus of expert opinion, particularly in areas where the evidence is deficient and where policy makers are also involved.

The Current Situation

The current situation with regard to the implementation of research findings relating to the detection, assessment, diagnosis and monitoring of caries to ensure optimal *personalized caries management,* including clinical prevention and caries control in dental practice, is variable. In some countries implementation has been successful for many years and preventive caries control with a focus on the timely management of initial lesions is seen as established practice and is not controversial [2]. Effective adoption of evidence-based caries control has been seen in the Scandinavian countries for some decades and the Nexo model is an impressive example of what can be achieved [7]. This study assessed the effectiveness of a non-operative caries treatment programme used since 1987 in the municipality of Nexo in Denmark. The mean DMFS among 18-year-olds in 1999/2000 showed that children moving to adulthood in Nexo had significantly less caries than in the comparison municipalities [7]. Recent examples also include efforts in Colombia and elsewhere in South America to adopt the ICDAS approach in clinical practice as well as in education.

In a number of other countries, it is at the implementation step where the adoption of preventive caries control exploiting careful detection, assessment, diagnosis and monitoring of caries seems to have failed [2]. Despite what is taught in contemporary dental education, the general dental practice community is often still focussed around the restorative/surgical management of caries, which is still the basis of many remuneration systems. Often in these environments, no clinical value is seen in assessing lesions prior to the obvious cavitation stage.

In terms of failure to implement research findings, a further example is around attempts to clinically remineralize caries lesions. An International Conference on Novel Anticaries and Remineralizing Agents, held in 2008, reviewed existing evidence on caries remineralization within the context of 'modern' clinical management of the caries process aiming to prevent progression by promoting arrest and, where possible, regression of precavitation lesions. The delegates concluded that, as much of the evidence reviewed has been published but not adopted for decades, programmes for more effective dissemination and implementation of research findings with educators, clinicians and patients are required [8].

There is a need to better understand the different degrees of success in implementing cariology evidence to dentists in different countries. This is also important in terms of the mismatch between what students are taught in modern dental education and the reality students face when they graduate.

Opportunities for Implementation

The position regarding the current state of the evidence and international consensus is outlined in earlier chapters according to the framework shown in figure 2. This 'flow chart' for ICDAS-enabled, patient-centred caries management identifies the key steps which should be taken into consideration for implementation. This should be done in a flexible and locally appropriate way that still follows where the evidence leads and can be updated as new findings are added to synthesized knowledge in the specific areas covered.

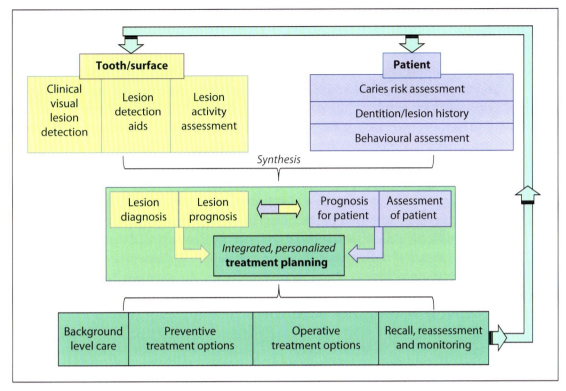

Fig. 2. The clinical framework for implementing ICDAS-enabled, patient-centred caries management.

It is hoped that bringing the information together in the form of a book will aid this implementation process for some. It is timely to address the implementation issue as we now have a distilled view from the research community on many aspects of the detection, assessment, diagnosis and monitoring of caries [9], as well as a structure seeking to facilitate the lines of communication between caries epidemiology, research and appropriate clinical management [1]. This information, e-learning packages in a number of languages and updated ICDAS research [10] are now available from the World Wide Web, as are primary research papers.

Implementation opportunities can be considered under each of the dental domains, but with a focus here on clinical practice.

Clinical Practice

At a governmental level, there is now an opportunity to capitalize on the World Health Organization's global policy for improvement of oral health, which follows on from the Sixtieth World Health Assembly of 2007 which adopted an action plan for health promotion and *integrated disease prevention* [11]. It states that when framing policies and strategies for oral health, particular emphasis should be laid on 'building of capacity in oral-health systems oriented to disease prevention and primary health care' and that 'oral-health services should be set up, ranging from prevention, early diagnosis and intervention to provision of treatment and rehabilitation, and the management of oral health problems of the population according to needs and to resources available'.

This links well with the International Dental Federation's promotion of minimally invasive dentistry [12] and initial work undertaken by the American Dental Association reviewing caries classification systems.

At the dental practice level there are a range of opportunities in many countries to link these developments to patients' preferences and the wider moves towards well-being and health, and health maintenance. This type of oral care is being seen as a practice builder and, compared to operative dentistry and local anaesthesia, is giving patients what they want from modern dentistry. There is also a good fit with the changes in skill mix seen in many countries – moving towards the dentist, in a number of situations, becoming more of an oral physician leading oral health teams focussed on prevention and disease control [2].

Epidemiology/Public Health

There have been an increasing number of epidemiological surveys being reported with the inclusion of lesions seen by clinical visual examination within the enamel as well as those in the dentine. A notable example is the most recent National Child Dental Health Survey carried out in Iceland which used ICDAS criteria [Agustsdottir, pers. commun.]. The data produced from such surveys should more closely match the planning needs for the types of preventive as well as restorative dental services being commissioned and delivered than do the traditional estimates just recording cavities to be filled. The availability of e-learning aids to examiner training also assists implementation [10]. Activities across the European Union have moved towards using the approach of including initial lesions in epidemiological surveys [13] and also making use of health surveillance opportunities by gathering ICDAS data from general dentists [14].

Research

Having now identified a series of research priorities in this field, the opportunity to drive forward research and innovation in the areas where we need them is clear to researchers, research funding agencies and the oral health industry and its partners.

There are a number of existing and developing international collaborations active in this area within the caries research community. Particular interest is being shown in the widening open system of the ICDAS, working alongside and with networks of researchers within the European Organization for Caries Research, and the International Association for Dental Research.

Education

In dental education some years ago, Kidd and Fejerskov [15] issued a challenge to dental schools to accept responsibility for changing the attitude of dental practitioners to reflect modern evidence in cariology and, in particular, to recognize that efforts to arrest lesion progression and prevent cavity development were a clinical priority. In recent years there seems to be a response to this call from some of those countries where the misalignment between education and practice continued. Opportunities include: the sharing of resource materials, as in the creation of the ICDAS e-learning package [10]; the plans for a European curriculum in cariology brokered by the European Organization for Caries Research and the Association for Dental Education in Europe, and the creation of a Cariology Special Interest Group within the American Dental Education Association. In Australia there have been widespread moves towards adopting minimally invasive dentistry in practice, and this is mirrored by the development of an evidence-based preventive strategy for dental practitioners which is also taught in the dental school setting [16].

Challenges to Implementation

Implementation challenges can be considered under each of the dental domains, but again with a focus here on clinical practice.

Clinical Practice

The interventive and restorative philosophy underlying many dental payment systems has been identified as a fundamental barrier to the adoption of more holistic and preventive caries management strategies by many authors and authorities. This is a serious challenge which needs urgent and imaginative solutions from all those involved, including the professional associations. In a number of the earlier chapters, specific barriers to implementation have been identified, and these should all be addressed where they are relevant to a specific country or practice.

What is remarkable is that the teachings of an iconic dentist, Dr. G.V. Black, should still hold so much sway 100 years after his key texts on restorative caries management were published. Without going into detail, it seems clear that Black, a keen and observant researcher, might now be horrified if he were still alive and learn that the use of evidence had not moved on from what was known 100 years ago. Black wrote on the importance of enamel caries and sought to provide preventive and long-lasting care for his patients. There is a dissemination gap regarding cariology findings and their clinical relevance to many general dentists. This allows attitudes to persist in which it is clear that many practising dentists focus only on restorative caries care. Unfortunately this position is attracting the attention of others, such as those writing in a recent editorial for physicians in *The Lancet* that dentists are not embracing prevention [17].

Evans et al. [16] cite as 'one of the main reasons for the current attitude' among those still focussing on restorative-only caries management the confusion that is created by terminology and the use of the term 'dental caries' to represent both the disease and its manifestation. The 'Glossary of key terms' set out in the next chapter seeks to address this important but neglected issue.

Epidemiology/Public Health

In epidemiology and dental public health there are still many 'traditionalists' who appear to be wedded to the past in terms of methodology, and some seem stuck in a straightjacket of making solely retrospective comparisons with never changing criteria or methods. There are communication issues to overcome in understanding that caries data can be collected at a detailed level and then, in parallel, recalculated in software to compute estimates of what would have been reported if earlier conventions had been followed. There are also apparently updating and continuing education challenges to ensure that all are kept up to date with cariology as a discipline and current best evidence. This is problematic for those commissioning and evaluating clinical caries-preventive interventions.

Research

There have been threats to caries research for some decades in terms of securing funding for this subject area at a time when the continuing burden and long-term societal costs of the disease [11, 17] were not well understood in many countries. This is a continuing issue which should be addressed by research funding organizations.

Education

There are serious concerns in a number of countries that, as a cohort of 'cariologists' retire, many are not being replaced by junior faculty teaching and researching in the area. This is a real threat when it is increasingly recognized that it is vital to communicate up-to-date scientific and clinical knowledge about dental caries to undergraduate and graduate dentists, as well as to the wider oral health care and health care teams.

The Future

If there are to be sustainable improvements made in delivering what we currently have, as well as further improvement made to the detection, assessment, diagnosis and monitoring of caries to ensure optimal personalized caries management, then some of the disparate activities outlined above will have to be tackled and brought more into alignment.

Figure 1, with the Collaboration for Improving Dentistry model, shows how the various processes around evidence creation and synthesis need to be more closely and systematically synchronized with dissemination of findings to all stakeholders and the education community. It also shows the most difficult challenge to be overcome: implementation to make a difference to the clinician-patient interaction. This last element needs to be a much clearer focus in the future for all who seek to improve caries care for patients. In the future, what are sometimes in clinical cariology the discrete 'silos' of clinical practice, epidemiology/public health, research and education will have to communicate better and work more closely together if any of these domains are going to truly realize their potential contributions to oral health.

As was pointed out in the chapter by Pitts [this vol., pp. 1–14], it is also important to realize that the clinical focus taken for this book should in no way detract from the parallel ICDAS missions going forward (which are to lead to better-quality information to influence decisions about the appropriate diagnosis, prognosis and clinical management at both the individual and public health levels) in the domains of dental public health/epidemiology, clinical research or dental education.

Figure 2 uses the ICDAS-enabled, patient-centred caries management framework to identify the key steps which have to be addressed in a locally sensitive way for optimal implementation. This framework is iterative, and there needs to be an increased focus on longitudinal care and long-term treatment planning. The framework should also drive the research agenda in the area.

In the future the dental community should implement the evidence it has in the detection, assessment, diagnosis and monitoring of caries to ensure optimal personalized caries management and move towards innovative new caries control and remineralization methods that work in formats that are acceptable in all parts of the world. It is important that in caries control we 'short-circuit' the painful learnings of some 'western' dental societies and, for emerging countries move straight to an integrated secondary preventive model, linked to primary prevention and also to working with other professions and agencies for a maximal impact on oral health and health in general.

The broadly agreed future research agenda arising from the International Conference on Novel Anticaries and Remineralizing Agents [8] is also relevant here and fits into the framework in figure 2. This group recognized that the aim is to facilitate caries control over a lifetime using evidence-based, clinically effective, multifactorial prevention to keep the caries process in balance. Over the coming years the dental research community in this field should continue to apply new knowledge and methods from outside dentistry and develop a menu of caries control strategies effective for individuals, groups and populations using agreed, comparable protocols.

A new and important focus for the future should also be research into *getting research findings into routine practice, with impacts on the behaviour of patients, professionals and policy makers*. This agenda of type 2 and 3 translational research is required if we are to understand in the future how best to get cariology research findings implemented in routine clinical practice.

References

1 Pitts NB: 'ICDAS' – an international system for caries detection and assessment being developed to facilitate caries epidemiology, research and appropriate clinical management. Community Dent Health 2004;21:193–198.
2 Pitts NB: Are we ready to move from operative to non-operative/preventive treatment of dental caries in clinical practice? Caries Res 2004;38:294–304.
3 Pitts NB: Understanding the jigsaw of evidence based dentistry. 1. Introduction, research and synthesis. J Evid Based Dent 2004;5:2–4.
4 Pitts NB: Understanding the jigsaw of evidence based dentistry. 2. Dissemination of research results. J Evid Based Dent 2004;5:33–35.
5 Pitts NB: Understanding the jigsaw of evidence based dentistry. 3. Implementation of research findings. J Evid Based Dent 2004;5:60–64.
6 Bonetti D, Pitts NB, Eccles M, Grimshaw J, Johnston M, Steen N, Shirran E, Thomas R, MacLennan G, Clarkson JE, Walker A: Applying psychological theory to evidence-based practice: identifying factors predictive to taking intra-oral radiographs. Soc Sci Med 2006;63:1889–1899.
7 Ekstrand KR, Christiansen MEC: Outcomes of a non-operative caries treatment programme for children and adolescents. Caries Res 2005;39:455–467.
8 Pitts NB, Wefel JS: Remineralization/desensitization: what is known now and what is the future? Adv Dent Res, 2009, in press.
9 Pitts NB, Stamm J: International Consensus Workshop on Caries Clinical Trials (ICW-CCT) – final consensus statements: agreeing where the evidence leads. J Dent Res 2004;83(spec iss C):125–128.
10 ICDAS – International Caries Detection and Assessment System. www.icdas.org.
11 Petersen P-E: World Health Organization global policy for improvement of oral health – World Health Assembly 2007. Int Dent J 2008;58:115–121.
12 Tyas MJ, Anusavice KJ, Frencken JE, Mount GJ: Minimal intervention dentistry – a review. FDI Commission Project 1-97. Int Dent J 2000;50:1–12.
13 European Association of Dental Public Health. www.eadph.org/.
14 Bourgeois DM, Christensen LB, Ottolenghi L, Llodra JC, Pitts NB, Senakola E (eds): Health Surveillance in Europe – European Global Oral Health Indicators Development Project Oral Health Interviews and Clinical Surveys: Guidelines. Lyon, Lyon I University Press, 2008.
15 Kidd EAM, Fejerskov O: Prevention of dental caries and the control of disease progression: concepts of preventive nonoperative treatment; in Fejerskov O, Kidd EAM (eds): Dental Caries – The Disease and Its Clinical Management. Oxford, Blackwell Munksgaard, 2003, pp 167–169.
16 Evans RW, Pakdaman A, Dennison PJ, Howe ELC: The Caries Management System: an evidence-based preventive strategy for dental practitioners – application for adults. Aust Dent J 2008;53:83–92.
17 Editorial – oral health: prevention is key. Lancet 2009;373:1.

N.B. Pitts
Dental Health Services and Research Unit, University of Dundee
Mackenzie Building, Kirsty Semple Way
Dundee DD2 4BF (UK)
Tel. +44 1382 420067, Fax +44 1382 420051, E-Mail n.b.pitts@cpse.dundee.ac.uk

Glossary of Key Terms

C. Longbottom[a] · M.-C. Huysmans[b] · N.B. Pitts[a] · M. Fontana[c]

[a]Dental Health Services and Research Unit, University of Dundee, Dundee, UK; [b]Department of Cariology & Endodontology, TRIKON: Institute for Dental Clinical Research, University of Nijmegen, Nijmegen, The Netherlands; [c]Department of Preventive and Community, Dentistry Oral Health Research Center, Indiana University School of Dentistry, Indianapolis, Ind., USA

Precision of word definition is a critical element in any scientific endeavour; it is also essential in accurate and effective communication between clinicians and, separately, with patients. There exists a huge body of dental literature, spanning over a century, which constitutes the evolving scientific research into caries, cariology, and which is suffused with confusing and sometimes contradictory (explicit and implicit) definitions of numerous words. Within this cariology literature there is, unfortunately, even a range of uses for the word 'caries' itself [1]. This leads to ambiguity, misunderstanding and lack of scientific rigour within the literature, despite the best endeavours of cariology researchers and peer reviewers. Within the international dental community there is no single generally recognized authoritative body or group responsible for specifying (and maintaining) scientifically robust definitions in relation to caries.

Attempting to modify this situation presents a number of challenges, including addressing the well-recognized ambiguities present within the international scientific language – English – as well as translation issues relating to the existence of words in English which may not be readily translated into another particular language. Establishing an internationally recognized set of definitions in relation to caries will require agreement between and co-operation amongst a wide range of groups and individuals.

A number of consensus development conferences, national dental association committees, as well as other dental organizations, have variously attempted to address this problem by debating and developing definitions which reflect up-to-date evidence in relation to various specific aspects of caries. These initiatives include the International Consensus Workshop on Caries Clinical Trials conference in 2002 [2], which brought together 95 international experts from academia, industry and the regulatory community who came from 23 countries. Following 25 presentations of evidence overviews, in the format of an international consensus workshop, they crafted, debated and finalized consensus statements which agreed 'where the evidence leads'. A key statement in the area of caries terminology was the agreement that 'there is some confusion with the terminology employed in the literature around caries diagnosis (which should imply a human professional summation of all available data), lesion detection (which implies some objective method of determining whether or not disease is present) and lesion assessment (which aims to characterize or monitor a lesion, once it has been detected)' [2].

This glossary is an attempt to compile a set of definitions in relation to a limited number of key words commonly used in relation to cariology and caries 'diagnosis'. This is merely a 'core' set of words most relevant to this publication and central to understanding the disease and its clinical management.

Additional, expanded, versions are required to address (at least) the four recognized dental domains for the use of such terms – *clinical practice, clinical research, epidemiology/public health* and *education* – each of which have different needs. Definitions need to be:
- fairly short and sharp for both clinicians and patients;
- detailed and unambiguous for research use;
- specific and compatible with use for populations in epidemiology;
- broader and with more background context in education.

In addition, there are various 'localization' requirements to be meaningful to specific countries, although there are significant opportunities for the international harmonization of such key terms in an increasingly global village. In some cases there will also be the need for some accepted synonyms – the use of caries/carious in different countries is but one example which is used below.

This work of expanding a common glossary is in progress with representatives of the International Caries Detection and Assessment System, the European Organization for Caries Research, the European Association of Dental Public Health and the American Dental Education Association Cariology Special Interest Group. The input of these organizations to the glossary of key terms presented here is also gratefully acknowledged.

The glossary is not in alphabetical order of terms, but, because the caries process involves physical and temporal domains and is dynamic in nature, it starts with the disease itself and the caries process, and then moves through:
- definitions related to the lesion, its detection, assessment (characterization/description) and diagnosis;
- followed by considerations of severity/extent and surface status;
- followed by considerations of activity, lesion behaviour and prognosis.

The Disease, the Caries Process and High-Level Terms

Dental Caries, the Disease

Dental caries is the localized destruction of susceptible dental hard tissue by acidic by-products from bacterial fermentation of dietary carbohydrates.

(This definition has been used in a recent *Lancet* review on dental caries [3] and reflects a synthesis of international evidence, including that presented from both basic and clinical cariology [4] as well as microbiology perspectives [5].)

Caries Process

The caries process is the dynamic sequence of biofilm-tooth interactions which can occur over time on and within a tooth surface.

(These bacteriochemical interactions may result in some or all of the complete spectrum – or stages – of damage, ranging from initial outer surface demineralization, at the molecular level, through subsurface demineralization producing enamel white-spot lesion formation, through macroscopic lesion cavitation, to dentine and pulpal infection, to complete tissue destruction. Relentless progression through all these stages of disease severity is *not* inevitable.)

Caries Lesion/Carious Lesion

A caries/carious lesion is a detectable change in the tooth structure that results from the biofilm-tooth interactions occurring due to the disease caries.

(These interactions cause changes in the tooth mineral structure as well as in the much less plentiful organic parts of tooth structures.)

Caries/Carious Lesion Detection

A process [2] involving the recognition (and/or recording), traditionally by optical or physical means, of changes in enamel and/or dentine and/or cementum, which are consistent with having been caused by the caries process.

Caries/Carious Lesion Assessment

The evaluation of the characteristics [2] of a caries lesion, once it has been detected. These characteristics may include optical, physical, chemical or biochemical parameters, such as colour, size or surface integrity.

Caries Diagnosis

The human professional summation of all the signs and symptoms of disease [2] to arrive at an identification of the past or present occurrence of the disease caries.

Assessment of Caries Lesions

Caries Lesion Severity

The stage of lesion progression along the spectrum of net mineral loss, from the initial loss at a molecular level to total tissue destruction. This involves elements of both the extent of the lesion in a pulpal direction and the mineral loss in volume terms.

Caries Lesion (Pulpal) Extent

A physical measurement/assessment of the net mineral loss in a pulpal direction. This can be graded, scaled or measured as fractions of enamel and/or dentine thickness, in a pulpal direction, which have undergone net mineral loss.

White-Spot Lesion

A caries/carious lesion which has reached the stage where the net subsurface mineral loss has produced changes in the optical properties of enamel such that these are visibly detectable as a loss of translucency, resulting in a white appearance of the enamel surface.

Brown-Spot Lesion

A caries/carious lesion which has reached the stage where the net subsurface mineral loss in conjunction with the acquisition of intrinsic or exogenous pigments has produced changes in the optical properties of enamel such that these are visibly detectable as a loss of translucency and a brown discolouration, resulting in a brown appearance of the enamel surface.
   (This should be differentiated from superficial stain.)

Non-Cavitated Lesion

A caries/carious lesion whose surface appears macroscopically to be intact.

Microcavity/Microcavitation

A caries/carious lesion with a surface which has lost its original contour/integrity, without clinicovisually distinct cavity formation.

(This may take the form of localized 'widening' of the enamel fissure morphology beyond its original features, within an initial enamel lesion, and/or a very small cavity with no detectable dentine at the base.)

Cavity/Cavitated Lesion

A caries/carious lesion with a surface which is not macroscopically intact, with a distinct discontinuity or break in the surface integrity, as determined using optical or tactile means.

Caries Activity, Lesion Behaviour and Prognosis

Demineralization

The loss of calcified material from the structure of the tooth. This chemical process can be biofilm mediated – i.e. as in caries – or chemically mediated – i.e. as in erosion – from exogenous or endogenous sources of acid – e.g. from the diet, environment or stomach.

Remineralization

The net gain of calcified material within the tooth structure, replacing that which was previously lost by demineralization.

Caries Lesion Activity (Net Progression)

The summation of the dynamics of the caries process resulting in the net loss, over time, of mineral from a caries lesion – i.e. there is active lesion progression.

(Although a caries lesion which is undergoing net remineralization is in a state of chemical 'activity' – i.e. it is undergoing change and is therefore not chemically static –, the above definition is designed specifically to avoid possible confusion and register the clinical reality of a lesion in a state of disease progression, as opposed to disease regression.)

Active Caries Lesion

A caries lesion, from which, over a specified period of time, there is net mineral loss, i.e. the lesion is progressing.

[This may be identified by either: (a) a 1-point-in-time characterization of the lesion, using particular lesion parameters indicative of lesion progression, or (b) a comparison, at 2 or more time points, of specific lesion parameters/characteristics when monitoring a lesion.]

Caries/Carious Lesion Behaviour

Lesion behaviour is defined in terms of what changes, if any, occur in the status of a lesion over time in response to the balance between demineralization and remineralization.

[A lesion can, between 2 time points: (a) progress (exhibit net mineral loss), (b) arrest, i.e. remains unchanged (static/stable), or (c) regress (exhibit net mineral gain). At a further (third and/or subsequent) time point, the lesion can exhibit any of the above 3 changes, and hence can (d) undergo oscillations in status.]

Monitoring of a Caries/Carious Lesion

The assessment, over time, of one or more of the characteristics of a caries lesion to assess if any changes have occurred in that lesion.

[This can involve comparison of one or more of the characteristic(s), such as the severity or the extent or the activity of a lesion.]

Arrested or Inactive Caries Lesion

A lesion which is not undergoing net mineral loss – i.e. the caries process in a specific lesion is no longer progressing.

(This may be assessed by comparison/monitoring of lesion characteristics over a specified time period or by assessment/determination of lesion characteristics at a particular point in time, as being consistent with those of lesion arrest.)

Remineralized Caries Lesion

A caries lesion which exhibits evidence of having undergone net mineral gain – i.e. there is replacement of mineral which was previously lost due to the caries process.

Caries Lesion Regression

The net gain of calcified material to the structure of a caries lesion, replacing that which was previously lost by caries demineralization.

[This will involve a change in the area (2-dimensional) and/or volume (3-dimensional) of the mineral characteristics of the lesion and may lead to changes in mineral quality.]

Caries Lesion Prognosis

The likely future behaviour of (or clinical outcome for) a specific caries lesion, over a specified time period, as assessed by a clinician – taking into account the summation of the multiple factors impacting on the possible progression, arrest or regression of the lesion.

Clarified and Updated/Outmoded and Deprecated – Definitions and Terms

A number of forms of common dental 'usage' of some important caries-related terms persist from previous decades and these can serve to confuse. The confusion affects not only the dental community, but also the patients we serve, as well as the public and policy makers. Because of this confusion, in a number of cases it is important to clearly update definitions; in other cases it is no longer appropriate to use the term. Three examples are given below.

Minimally Invasive Dentistry

This is a vitally important term, but one which means different things to different people in dentistry. Its definition should be made clear.

(Minimally invasive dentistry is supported by the emerging evidence and international consensus, it has an international focus, from for example the Fédération Dentaire Internationale [6] and others [7], and continues to be built on. The approach of minimally invasive intervention stresses a preventive philosophy, individualized risk assessments, accurate, early detection of lesions and efforts to remineralize non-cavitated lesions with the prompt provision of preventive care in order to minimize operative intervention. When operative intervention is unequivocally required, typically for an active cavitated lesion, the procedure used should be as minimally invasive as possible.

What is not supported by the evidence or international consensus, but which is sometimes mislabelled as minimally invasive, is clinical activity in which small, early and inactive/arrested lesions are sought out and prematurely or unnecessarily subjected to operative intervention.)

Caries Free

This term has frequently been used when referring to assessments made (of either individuals or groups) even where the diagnostic threshold employed has been at the 'dentine or worse' level, ignoring all grades of initial lesion which may also be present. The term should now be avoided and more precise terms used.

(This term gives an erroneous impression that no disease is present and can readily confuse dentists, patients and policy makers [8]. In such circumstances, and also where lesion detection aids, such as radiographs, have not been used, the term 'no obvious dentine caries' is now preferred.)

Active Caries

This term used to be used to mean any lesion which had penetrated into dentine. The more modern definitions of 'activity' set out above should now be used.

(Some dentists, in the clinical practice or epidemiology domains, have traditionally used this term to describe any lesion in dentine, making no allowance for whether the lesion is actively progressing or is arrested.)

References

1 Evans RW, Pakdaman A, Dennison PJ, Howe ELC: The Caries Management System: an evidence-based preventive strategy for dental practitioners – application for adults. Aust Dent J 2008 53:83–92.
2 Pitts NB, Stamm J: International Consensus Workshop on Caries Clinical Trials (ICW-CCT) – final consensus statements: agreeing where the evidence leads. J Dent Res 2004;83(spec iss C):125–128.
3 Selwitz RH, Ismail AI, Pitts NB: Dental caries. Lancet 2007;369:51–59.
4 Fejerskov O, Kidd EAM (eds): Dental Caries: The Disease and Its Clinical Management. Copenhagen, Blackwell Munksgaard, 2003.
5 Marsh P, Martin MV: Oral Microbiology, ed 4. Oxford, Wright, 1999.
6 Tyas MJ, Anusavice KJ, Frencken JE, Mount GJ: Minimal intervention dentistry – a review. Int Dent J 2000;50:1–12.
7 Pitts NB: Are we ready to move from operative to non-operative/preventive treatment of dental caries in clinical practice? Caries Res 2004;38:294–304.
8 Pitts NB, Longbottom C: Preventive care advised (PCA)/operative care advised (OCA) – categorising caries by the management option. Community Dent Oral Epidemiol 1995;23:55–59.

C. Longbottom
Dental Health Services and Research Unit, University of Dundee
Mackenzie Building, Kirsty Semple Way
Dundee DD2 4BF (UK)
Tel. +44 1382 420064, Fax +44 1382 420051, E-Mail c.longbottom@cpse.dundee.ac.uk

Author Index

Amaechi, B.T. 188

Bonetti, D. 188

Clarkson, J.E. 188

Eggertsson, H. 102
Ekstrand, K.R. 63, 149, 156
Ellwood, R. 42, 52

Ferreira-Zandona, A. 102
Fontana, M. 91, 209
Freeman, R. 113

Huysmans, M.-C. 209

Ismail, A. 113

Kambara, M. 156

Longbottom, C. 52, 149, 156, 209
Lussi, A. 42, 52

Martignon, S. 63

Neuhaus, K.W. 42, 52
Ngo, H. 188

Pitts, N.B. 1, 15, 42, 63, 128, 144, 164, 174, 199, 209

Richards, D. 128
Ricketts, D.N.J. 164, 174

Topping, G.V.A. 15
Twetman, S. 91

Zero, D.T. 63, 149, 156

Subject Index

Active caries, definition 216
Active caries lesion
　definition 63, 214
　diagnostic approaches 64
　examples 64
　patho-anatomical features
　　primary coronal caries 66, 67
　　primary root caries lesions 68, 69
Air abrasion, caries removal 175, 176
Amalgam, trends in use 169, 170
Approximal sealants, preventive treatment 157
Arrested caries lesion
　definition 214, 215
　lesion arrest versus remineralization 108, 109
　patho-anatomical features
　　primary coronal caries 66, 67
　　primary root caries lesions 68, 69

Background level care (BLC)
　caries risk status change 147
　implementation considerations 148
　incorrect lesion assessment/diagnosis impact 147
　overview 146, 147
　research prospects 148
Behavior, see Caries lesion behavior; Patient behavior
Bitewing radiography
　diagnostic quality factors 44, 45
　digital versus film images 45, 46
　example 43
　frequency 46
　interpretation 46, 47
　treatment decisions 47
Black's cavity classification 165–169

Brown-spot lesion, definition 212, 213

Calcium phosphate, remineralization promotion 158
Caries cube, concept 5, 6, 145, 146
Caries diagnosis, definition 212
Caries free, definition 216
Caries lesion, definition 211
Caries lesion activity
　assessment, see Caries lesion assessment
　definition 214
　prospects for study 87
Caries lesion assessment
　definition 212
　gingival status 71
　patho-anatomical features
　　primary coronal caries 66, 67
　　primary root caries lesions 68, 69
　plaque
　　presence 69, 71
　　stagnation 70, 71
　reliability and accuracy studies of scoring systems
　　clinical studies 78–82
　　in vitro studies 73, 76
　　overview 72–75
　　root caries lesions 82, 83
　susceptibility determinants 72
Caries lesion behavior, definition 214
Caries lesion detection, see also International Caries Detection and Assessment System
　definition 211
　novel detection aids
　　electronic caries monitor 58, 59
　　laser fluorescence 52–55
　　quantitative light-induced fluorescence 55–57

subtraction radiography 57, 58
traditional detection aids
bitewing radiography 43–48
fiber-optic transillumination 49, 50
probing 42, 54
visual detection systems 15, 16
Caries lesion extent, definition 212
Caries lesion prognosis, definition 215
Caries lesion regression, definition 215
Caries lesion severity, definition 212
Caries management by risk assessment (CAMBRA) 133, 134
Carisolv, chemomechanical caries removal 175
Carlogram program 99
Cavity, *see also* Operative treatment
Black's classification
cavity design 167–169
overview 165, 166
definition 213
Collaboration for Improving Dentistry model 200, 201

Deep caries, management 178, 179
Demineralization, definition 213
Dental caries, definition 66, 211
Dentine, changes in primary coronal caries 67
Diagnodent, caries removal 178

Early childhood carrier (ECC)
definition 104
patterns in primary dentition 104
Electronic caries monitor (ECM)
modes 58
principles 58
root caries detection 59
Enamel
changes in primary coronal caries 66, 67
hypoplasia 108
laser treatment 159, 160
Enamelon, remineralization promotion 158
Eruption time
permanent molar eruption time and caries 106
primary dentition caries patterns 104
risk assessment 97

Fiber-optic transillumination (FOTI), caries lesion detection 49, 50
Fissure sealants, retention rate 180

Fluoride
application with slow-release fluoride devices 157, 158
caries lesion impact 84, 85

Gingiva, status and lesion activity assessment 71

Hall technique, *see* Preformed metal crowns
Health behavior, *see* Patient behavior
Health belief model (HBM) 114–116

International Caries Detection and Assessment System (ICDAS)
applications
clinical practice 19, 20
clinical research 12, 20
education 11, 20, 21
epidemiology 10, 11, 21
clinical framework for management implementation 6, 8, 9
codes
restoration status
caries adjacent to restorations and sealants 30, 31
Code 0 33
Code 1 34
Code 2 34
Code E 33
overview 22, 23
root caries 31–33
severity codes
Code 0 24, 25
Code 1 24, 26, 27
Code 2 26, 27
Code 3 27–29
Code 4 28, 29
Code 5 28–30
Code 6 30, 31
overview 23, 24
stages 23
codes and traditional prevention options
0–6 years 160
6–12 years 151
12–20 years 152
20 years and up 163
comparison with World Health Organization system 37, 38
examination
conditions 21, 22
outside clinic 22, 23

Subject Index

International Caries Detection and Assessment System (ICDAS) (continued)
  framework 129–131
  historical perspective 16–18
  lesion-related information 135–138
  Mount-Hume classification reconciliation 166–168
  overview 3, 4
  patient-related information 138, 139
  personalized caries management implementation, see Personalized caries management
  prospects
    implementation priorities 39
    research priorities 38
  reproducibility, sensitivity, and specificity 34–37
  treatment plan incorporation 129–131, 139–141
  vision 129

KAB model 113

Laser cavity reparation 177
Laser fluorescence (LF), caries lesion detection 52–55

Microcavity, definition 213
Minimally invasive dentistry
  definition 215, 216
  historical perspective 169
  tunnel preparation 170, 171
Motivational interviewing
  components 120, 121
  phase 1 121, 122
  phase 2 122
  phase 3 122
  phase 4 123
  phase 5 123

Non-cavitated lesion, definition 213
Novamin, remineralization promotion 158

Operative treatment
  air abrasion 175, 176
  Black's principle of cavity design 167–169
  caries removal extent
    fissure sealant studies 180
    novel approaches 177, 178
    stepwise evacuation 181–183

  systematic review of complete versus ultraconservative removal 183–185
  traditional treatment 171, 172, 179
  ultraconservative caries removal 180, 181
Carisolv and chemomechanical caries removal 175
composite resin use impact on cavity design 170
deep caries 178, 179
indications 164, 165
International Caries Detection and Assessment System classification of lesions 165–168
laser cavity reparation 177
polymer rotary burs 176
restorative materials 169, 170
sono-abrasion 176
tunnel preparation 170, 171
Ozone therapy, preventive treatment 159

Patient behavior
  assessment targets and professional assumptions 118, 119
  behavior change promotion
    motivational interviewing
      components 120, 121
      phase 1 121, 122
      phase 2 122
      phase 3 122
      phase 4 123
      phase 5 123
    overview 119, 120
    transtheoretical model
      action and maintenance 125
      components 123, 124
      contemplation 124, 125
      precontemplation 124
      preparation 125
      relapse 125, 126
  health behavior definition 114, 115
  KAB model 113
  models
    health belief model 114–116
    theory of planned behavior 116
    self-efficacy theory 117
  need concepts 117, 118
Patterns, caries
  caries experience effects 105, 106
  cavitated versus non-cavitated lesions 107
  enamel hypoplasia effects 108

eruption stage effects 105
lesion arrest versus remineralization 108, 109
malocclusion effects 108
permanent dentition 105
permanent molar eruption time effects 106
primary dentition 104
speed of progression 107
tooth surface susceptibility 106, 107
Personalized caries management
 Collaboration for Improving Dentistry model 200, 201
 current situation 201, 202
 evidence-based dentistry 200
 implementation via International Caries Detection and Assessment System
  opportunities
   clinical practice 203, 204
   education 205
   epidemiology/public health 204
   overview 202, 203
   research 204, 205
  challenges
   clinical practice 205, 206
   education 206
   epidemiology/public health 206
   research 206
  prospects 207, 208
 overview 199, 200
 translational medicine types 200, 208
 treatment planning, see Treatment planning
Plaque, lesion activity assessment
 presence 69, 71
 stagnation 70, 71
Polymer rotary burs, caries removal 176
Preformed metal crowns (PMCs)
 outcomes 184, 185
 preventive treatment 160
Preventive treatments
 approximal sealants 157
 calcium phosphate for remineralization promotion 158
 classification 150
 fluoride application with slow-release fluoride devices 157, 158
 implementation priorities 154, 162
 International Caries Detection and Assessment System codes and traditional prevention options
  0–6 years 160
  6–12 years 151

  12–20 years 152
  20 years and up 163
 laser treatment of enamel 159, 160
 novel approaches to preventive practice 160, 161
 ozone therapy 159
 preformed metal crowns 160
 prevention categories 149, 150, 156
 probiotics 159
 research prospects 153, 154, 162
 restorative cycle/spiral 152, 154
 Scottish Clinical Effectiveness Program classification of recommendation levels 152
Probing, caries lesion detection 42, 54
Probiotics, preventive treatment 159

Quantitative light-induced fluorescence (QLF), caries lesion detection 55–57

Radiography, see Bitewing radiography; Subtraction radiography
Recaldent, remineralization promotion 158
Recall system
 checklist of modifying factors for risk assessment 192–195
 function 188, 189
 positive impact 189
 recall interval recommendations 192, 194
 research prospects 196, 197
 United Kingdom experience 190–197
Remaining dentine thickness (RDT)
 deep caries management 178
 measurement 179
Remineralization
 definition 213
 lesion arrest versus remineralization 108, 109
Remineralized caries lesion, definition 215
Risk, definition 91
Risk assessment, caries
 checklist of modifying factors 192–195
 longitudinal trials
  findings
   posteruptive age effects 97
   root caries in adults 97, 98
   schoolchildren and adolescents 97
   toddlers and preschool children 95–97
  overview 95

Risk assessment, caries (continued)
  prospects for study 99
  terminology 94, 95
Risk factors, caries 92–94
Root caries
  activity assessment 82, 83
  electronic caries monitor detection 59
  patho-anatomical features in primary root caries lesions 68, 69
  risk assessment in adults 97, 98

Scottish Dental Clinical Effectiveness Program (SDCEP)
  grading scheme of recommendations 10, 11
  recommendation levels for preventive treatments 152
Sealants, *see* Approximal sealants; Fissure sealants
Self-efficacy theory 117
Smartprep, caries removal 176
Sono-abrasion, caries removal 176
SS White, caries removal 176
Stepwise evacuation, caries 181–183
Streptococcus mutans
  colonization of mouth 103
  prevention of colonization 103, 104
Subtraction radiography, caries lesion detection 57, 58
Surgery, *see* Operative treatment

Theory of planned behavior (TPB) 116
Transtheoretical model (TTM)
  action and maintenance 125
  components 123, 124
  contemplation 124, 125
  precontemplation 124
  preparation 125
  relapse 125, 126
Treatment planning
  clinical framework for implementation 6, 8, 9
  comprehensive treatment 3
  evolution 129–131
  importance 132
  International Caries Detection and Assessment System
    framework 129–131
    lesion-related information 135–138
    patient-related information 138, 139
    planning 139–141
  personalized treatment planning developments
    United Kingdom 132, 133
    United States 133–135
    implementation issues 142
    research issues 141
Tunnel preparation, minimally invasive dentistry 170, 171

Visual detection, *see* Caries lesion detection

White-spot lesion, definition 212
World Health Assembly, oral health action plan 2
World Health Organization (WHO), caries detection and assessment system 37, 38